Practicing Neurology

Practicing Neurology

What You Need to Know, What You Need to Do

Rahman Pourmand, M.D.

Associate Professor, Department of Neurology, Indiana University School of Medicine and Indiana University Hospital, Indianapolis

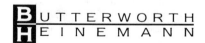

Boston   Oxford   Auckland   Johannesburg   Melbourne   New Delhi

Every effort has been made to ensure that the drug dosage schedules within this text are accurate and conform to standards accepted at time of publication. However, as treatment recommendations vary in the light of continuing research and clinical experience, the reader is advised to verify drug dosage schedules herein with information found on product information sheets. This is especially true in cases of new or infrequently used drugs.

All contents of this handbook represent the opinion of the author and do not reflect the official policy of the American Academy of Neurology or the institution with which the author is affiliated, unless this is clearly specified.

∞ Recognizing the importance of preserving what has been written, Butterworth–Heinemann prints its books on acid-free paper whenever possible.

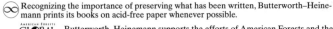 Butterworth–Heinemann supports the efforts of American Forests and the Global ReLeaf program in its campaign for the betterment of trees, forests, and our environment.

Library of Congress Cataloging-in-Publication Data

Pourmand, Rahman.
    Practicing neurology : what you need to know, what you need to do
/ Rahman Pourmand.
        p.   cm.
    Includes index.
    ISBN 0-7506-9970-1
    1. Neurology--Handbooks, manuals, etc.   2. Nervous system-
-Diseases--Handbooks, manuals, etc.   3. Nervous system--Diseases-
-Diagnosis--Handbooks, manuals, etc.   I. Title.
    [DNLM: 1. Nervous System Diseases--diagnosis.   2. Nervous System
Diseases--therapy.   WL 140 P877p 1999]
RC355.P68 1999
616.8--dc21
DNLM/DLC
    for Library of Congress   98-54985
                                                                          CIP

British Library Cataloguing-in-Publication Data
A catalogue record for this book is available from the British Library.

The publisher offers special discounts on bulk orders of this book.
For information, please contact:

Manager of Special Sales   For information on all
Butterworth–Heinemann   Butterworth–Heinemann publications
225 Wildwood Avenue   available, contact our World Wide Web
Woburn, MA 01801-2041   home page at http://www.bh.com
Tel: 781-904-2500
Fax: 781-904-2620

10 9 8 7 6 5 4 3 2 1

Printed in the United States of America

To Forough, Pejman, Mojgan, and Kamron

Contents

Preface   *ix*
Acknowledgments   *xi*

I. Evaluation   **1**
1. Highlights of Neurologic History and Examination   3
2. Neurologic Formulation   51
3. Neurologic Signs of Interest   53
4. Approach to the Patient with Suspected
   Hysteric Conversion   59
5. Neuroanatomy of Localization   63
6. Common Neurologic Constructs   67
7. Neurodiagnostic Tests and Procedures   79

II. Common Neurologic Conditions   **111**
8. Stroke   113
9. Seizure and Epilepsy   135
10. Central Nervous System Infections   145
11. Alteration of Mental Status   153
12. Demyelinating Disorders   163
13. Neurologic Complications of Alcohol   179
14. Dizziness and Vertigo   183
15. Primary Headaches and Facial Pain   189
16. Peripheral Neuropathy   209
17. Movement Disorders   223
18. Sleep Disorders   235
19. Neuromuscular Diseases   247
20. Back and Neck Pain   283

III. Neurologic Urgencies and Emergencies   **289**
21. Coma   291
22. Status Epilepticus   303
23. Brain Edema, Transtentorial Herniation,
    and Increased Intracranial Pressure   311

24. Metastatic Epidural Spinal Cord Compression   315
25. Acute Meningitis and Encephalitis   317
26. Delirium Tremens   321
27. Wernicke's Encephalopathy   325
28. Myasthenia Gravis Crisis   329
29. Guillain-Barré Syndrome   333
30. Temporal Arteritis   337

Index   *341*

Preface

When medical students and non-neurology residents rotating through the neurology service are asked about their expectations, their responses are uniform: They want to learn how to conduct effective neurologic examinations, they want to know the value and indications of neurologic procedures and testing, and they want to know how to evaluate and manage common neurologic conditions. This book addresses those topics.

After practicing neurology for almost 20 years in an academic setting, I believe I have met the expectations of my students, so I decided to put it in writing for others as well. In my opinion, knowing or reading thousands of pages of textbooks is not only impossible but also unnecessary to diagnose and treat the common neurologic conditions that physicians encounter in day-to-day practice, whether in the hospital, clinic, or emergency room. This book summarizes what and how much you need to know and do to confidently diagnose and manage most neurologic cases. You do not have to be a genius to figure out why a patient has footdrop. The bottom line is that neurology is not difficult; it just takes longer to do and requires mental exercises to reach the diagnosis. This handbook makes neurology easy, stimulating, and fun.

RP

Acknowledgments

I thank the faculty members in the Indiana University School of Medicine neurology department who reviewed the chapters and provided constructive criticism. I express my appreciation to Jennifer James and Linda Hagan for preparing the manuscript.

I am grateful to my publisher, Susan Pioli, and Assistant Editor Leslie Kramer, both of Butterworth–Heinemann, for their understanding, continued support, and patience. Last, I am indebted to a broad range of neurologic textbooks, handbooks, and papers in writing this book.

Acknowledgments

Practicing Neurology

Evaluation

1

Highlights of Neurologic History and Examination

GENERAL CONSIDERATIONS

The primary objective of medical students and residents rotating in neurology service is to be able to perform good neurologic examinations. They often think that the neurologic examination is difficult to remember and perform. I believe, however, that many medical students and junior residents do not know what to look for, how to find neurologic signs, and how to interpret their findings.

This chapter summarizes my views on and method of performing the neurologic examination. After practicing neurology for several years, I have found the methods described in this chapter to be useful, practical, and easy to remember. These views are by no means complete and standard, and I understand that some are subject to disagreement with other neurologists.

Despite expertise contained in more detailed text-books, there is no standard neurologic examination, and most neurologists develop their own techniques. I advise medical students and residents to examine the patient systematically, in an order they can remember.

I follow this sequence: mental status check, followed by tests of motor and sensory cranial nerves (CNs), including cerebellar reflexes and gait. Depending on the case, however, I may begin with the problem area first.

Although I recommend a systematic examination, flexibility also is important. A detailed neurologic examination is not always possible (e.g., in comatose or agitated patients or infants). To make the neurologic examination easier, unless clinically indicated, I do not routinely include several tests (e.g., smell test, Weber's and Rinne tests, gag reflex, taste test, corneal reflex, temperature). I see no reason to check the anal wink reflex in a patient complaining of headaches or the corneal reflex in a patient presenting with weakness. On the other hand, students should perform a complete neurologic examination to validate signs and variability and to gain confidence and experience. In cooperative, uncomplicated patients, a complete neurologic examination can be completed in 20–25 minutes.

The purpose of a neurologic examination, including taking a history, is to develop hypotheses about the nature and location of any lesion, to plan the investigation, and to set a course of therapy.

NEUROLOGIC HISTORY

Taking a thorough, detailed history is the most important part of the neurologic evaluation because the neurologic examination is based on the history. Listen to the patient carefully, and show that you are interested and concerned. A good strategy is to consider that the patient's history is indicative of an underlying neurologic disorder until proved otherwise. Remember that by history taking, you are checking most parts of the mental status examination. By asking the right questions, the following should be established:

- Likely anatomic sites (**Where is the lesion?**)
- Likely cause—vascular, neoplastic, infectious, or other (**What is the lesion?**)
- The onset of illness and temporal profile (e.g., acute, subacute, chronic, progressive, paroxysmal)

Remember: If you are not able to establish the above hypotheses after taking the history, do not pursue the neurologic examination. Go back and take more history.

After the history and physical examination are completed, follow up with the following:

- Consolidate pertinent findings and list differential diagnoses based on localization and etiologies.
- Plan the investigation and systematically order tests to confirm or support your hypothesis or to exclude others.

- Discuss the management and prognosis with the patient, and set a follow-up plan.

Most patients are unfamiliar with neurologic examinations; not only are neurologic examinations different from most physical examinations, they also are more complex and take longer. Communication with the patient during the examination is crucial. Explain what you are going to do, what you are trying to accomplish, and how the examination can help diagnose the problem. To gain the patient's trust and cooperation, pay early attention to the patient's problem, perhaps examining the problematic area first. If you decide to check the problem later in the examination, inform the patient.

The patient's comfort is important. For example, if the patient is supine, start with tests in that position (e.g., heel-to-shin test, abdominal reflexes, sensory testing, Babinski's sign). Proceed next to a sitting position and then to standing tests.

MENTAL STATUS AND HIGHER CORTICAL FUNCTION EXAMINATION

Before testing higher cortical function, you should establish that the patient is awake and alert, can hear, and is not aphasic. Higher cortical function testing is not necessary in all patients; for the most part, cognitive function can be assessed when taking the history. In this setting, I quickly check orientation, attention, short-term memory, judgment, and insight. I conduct formal higher function testing, however, if the patient complains of memory loss, is suspected of having dementia, or has a recent change in mental function or if I find a deficit or problem during the history taking.

What to Do

The Mini-Mental State Examination is used for bedside evaluation of cognitive function. In contrast to more detailed neuropsychometric testing, this test does not differentiate focal from diffuse central nervous system (CNS) lesions. The highest possible test score is 30 points; a patient who scores less than 23 has mental impairment.

Test	Score
Orientation	10
Retention and recall	6
Attention and calculation	5
Naming	2
Repetition	1
Comprehension	3
Reading and writing	2
Construction block	1

I check for **agnosia** and **apraxia** as part of the cognition test. Before testing for these abnormalities, verify that the patient can see and is able to touch and has no motor weakness or hand incoordination. Agnosia and apraxia can indicate parietal occipital lobe lesion. Note the presence of any of the following abnormalities:

- Inability to draw a clock or cross (construction apraxia)
- Inability to comb hair or drink through a straw (ideational apraxia)
- Inability to name fingers (finger agnosia)
- Inability to recognize objects by touch (astereognosis)
- Inability to recognize numbers drawn in hand (agraphesthesia)

Interpretation

A patient with deficits in several areas of the Mini-Mental State Examination has either a diffuse or multifocal CNS disorder. Chronic, slowly progressive problems may indicate dementing illness caused by a degenerative disorder. Acute or subacute problems may indicate confused state caused by toxic or metabolic derangement.

A patient who shows only a few deficits may have focal CNS insult. Look for additional focal signs, such as aphasia, visual field defect, and hemiparesis. A patient who demonstrates finger agnosia should be checked for dyscalculia, left-right disorientation, and dysgraphia, all of which are symptoms of Gerstmann's syndrome and indicative of a dominant parietal lobe lesion (stroke).

Caveat: The two most common causes of dementia are Alzheimer's disease and multiple strokes. Dementia can easily be mistaken for global confusion, depression (particularly in the elderly), aphasia, mental retardation, or psychiatric illness. Long-term memory loss with preserved short-term memory is clinically insignificant.

CRANIAL NERVE EXAMINATION

Anatomy

- All CNs except CNs I and II originate from the brain stem.
- The nuclei of CNs III and IV are located in the midbrain; the nuclei of CNs V, VII, and VIII are located in the pons; the nuclei of CNs IX, X, XI, and XII are located in the medulla.
- CNs I, II, and VIII are purely sensory; CNs III, IV, VI, XI, and XII are purely motor; the remainder are mixed.
- CNs III, VII, IX, and X have parasympathetic fibers.

Possible Sources of Cranial Nerve Dysfunction

- Supranuclear lesion
- Brain stem nuclei
- Nerve itself
- Neuromuscular junction
- Surrounding structures (e.g., cerebellum)

Some Clinical Hints

- CN dysfunction implies a lesion above the foramen magnum; therefore, spinal cord lesion does cause signs and symptoms of CN abnormalities.

- CN abnormalities plus ipsilateral appendicular motor or sensory deficits are consistent with supranuclear lesion (e.g., stroke).
- CN abnormalities plus contralateral, appendicular, motor, or sensory deficits indicate brain stem lesion (e.g., stroke, tumor).
- Unilateral dysfunction in CNs V, VI, VII, and VIII, plus contralateral appendicular motor or sensory deficit, suggests cerebellopontine angle lesion (e.g., tumor).
- Unilateral dysfunction of CN IX, X, or XI without appendicular deficit is seen in foramen jugular lesion (e.g., tumor).
- Unilateral abnormality of CN III, IV, or V suggests cavernous sinus lesion (e.g., thrombosis).
- Unilateral abnormality of CNs IX, XI, and XII indicates bulbar palsy (e.g., stroke).

Cranial Nerve I (Olfactory Nerve)

Most neurologists rarely test CN I; it is tested only if the patient complains of an olfactory problem. I usually ask the patient if he or she has difficulty smelling. When checking for smelling difficulties, examine each nostril separately by closing the other. Any scent can be used to test this nerve.

Clinical Hints

- Anosmia is absence of the sense of smell; hyposmia is diminished sense of smell.

- The sense of smell diminishes with increasing age.
- The most common causes of bilateral anosmia and hyposmia are the common cold and trauma to the nose.
- Neurologic diseases associated with hyposmia include Parkinson's disease, dementia, and vitamin B_{12} deficiency.
- Unilateral anosmia may indicate a subfrontal tumor.
- Hyposmia commonly is associated with difficulty in tasting.
- Ammonia is recognized through the trigeminal nerve (CN V); therefore, a patient who has no sense of smell, including of ammonia, may have a functional disorder (hysteric conversion).

Examination of the Eye (Cranial Nerves II, III, IV, and VI)

Neurologic examination of CNs II, III, IV, and VI includes checks of the following:

- Eyelids
- Pupils
- Visual acuity
- Visual field
- Fundi
- Eye movements

Examination of the eyes begins with the examiner sitting or standing in front of the patient (except when checking the pupillary light reflex). Note any eye globe asymmetry or droopy eyelids (ptosis).

What Does Ptosis Indicate?

- Isolated, fixed, unilateral ptosis usually is congenital or caused by an old eye trauma.
- Droopy eyelids on elderly patients may be caused by eyelid muscle laxity associated with age.
- Ptosis accompanied by abnormality of pupils may indicate Horner's syndrome or be caused by paralysis of the third nerve.
- Fluctuating, unilateral, or bilateral ptosis suggests myasthenia gravis. Ptosis should not be mistaken with eye closure weakness in Bell's palsy.

Pupils

Make note of the following irregularities when checking the pupils:

- Asymmetry of size or anisocoria
- Asymmetry of direct, consensual light reflex
- Irregularity of pupillary border

Pupillary eye examinations should include a check of pupillary reaction to accommodation and the swinging flashlight test.

Remember: The afferent pathway for pupillary light reflex is the optic nerve; for accommodation, it is the frontal lobes. The efferent pathway for both is the parasympathetic fibers of the third nerve. Examine the pupils in a semidark room. Stay by the patient's side (do not stand in front of the patient), and ask the patient to fixate on a distant object.

The following common pupillary abnormalities may be observed during examination:

- Anisocoria of up to 2 mm is a normal variant in pupils of an otherwise normal, awake person; it is abnormal (until proven otherwise) in an unconscious patient.
- Elderly individuals usually have smaller pupils.
- If one pupil does not constrict as compared with the other eye during the swinging flashlight test, the patient has **Marcus Gunn pupil**. Marcus Gunn pupil usually indicates an optic nerve lesion anterior to the chiasm, such as optic neuritis, and is always unilateral.
- **Horner's syndrome** consists of miosis, ptosis, and anhydrosis and can arise from any lesion from the hypothalamus to the superior cervical ganglion. The syndrome is commonly seen in neck pathologies. A cocaine and amphetamine test is used to differentiate a first-order neuron from a third-order neuron lesion.
- **Adie's pupil** is common in young, healthy women. One eye is dilated and has poor reaction to direct light. Some patients may have hyporeflexia on the same side (Adie-Holmes syndrome).

- **Argyll-Robertson pupils**, caused by a midbrain lesion, are small and bilateral with poor reaction to direct light, but adequate reaction to accommodation. Argyll-Robertson pupils are seen in syphilitic tabes and diabetes.

Visual Acuity

Check visual acuity (VA) in a well-lighted room. Always ask the patient if he or she uses glasses; if so, check VA with the glasses on. I use a near-vision chart held 30 mm from the patient. Check VA of each eye separately. Decreased VA with correction is seen in any ocular pathology and optic nerve lesion.

Visual Field

Visual field (VF) is divided vertically into nasal and temporal fields from the patient's point of view. VF defects are **homonymous** when the same part of the field is affected for both eyes; an exact match is **congruous**; no match is **incongruous**.

Different confrontation techniques can be used when making a VF evaluation, and each neurologist has strong opinions about technique. An evaluation should include the following basic checks. Sit or stand approximately 1 meter from the patient. Check each eye separately. Moving your fingers bilaterally helps detect **visual inattention**. Ask the patient to stare at a fixed point. With your hands apart and approximately 30 cm above the patient's eye level, hold up a number of fingers and ask the patient to count the fingers.

It is difficult to perform a VF evaluation of an uncooperative or lethargic patient. In these cases, check blink reflex to threat.

Common VF defects include the following:

- Tubular vision indicates nonorganic disease.
- Bitemporal hemianopia is caused by a chiasmatic lesion.
- Homonymous quadrantanopia is caused by a temporoparietal lobe lesion.
- Homonymous hemianopia, when **incongruous**, indicates an optic tract lesion; when it is **congruous**, it indicates a lesion behind the lateral geniculate body. **Macular sparing** indicates occipital cortex lesion.

Caveat: If a VF defect is limited to one eye, consider ocular, retinal, or optic nerve lesion; if the VF defect is bilateral, consider a lesion at or behind the chiasm or bilateral anterior to the chiasm.

Fundi

Fundoscopy should be done in all patients presenting with neurologic complaints. Dim the light and sit or stand in front of the patient. Ask the patient to stare at one spot on the wall. With your right hand holding the ophthalmoscope, check the right eye by approaching the eye from the right side at about a 15-degree angle; then repeat the procedure with the left hand holding the ophthalmoscope for the left eye. During fundoscopy, check the eye for retinal problems, blood vessel abnormalities, and optic discs. A basic knowledge of normal variants is essential (e.g., normal pigmentation on the disc edge, nasal blurriness, temporal pallor of the discs).

Remember: If the patient cannot see (decreased VA) but the disc margin is well defined, the patient likely has retrobulbar optic neuritis. If the patient cannot see (decreased VA) and the disc margin is not visible, consider optic neuritis or papillitis. If the patient sees well but the disc margin is not visible, papilledema is indicated. Optic neuritis and retrobulbar optic neuritis usually are unilateral; papilledema usually is bilateral.

Eye Movement (Cranial Nerves III, IV, and VI)

When checking eye movements or extraocular movements (EOMs), remain about an arm's length from the patient to avoid strain on convergence. Ask the patient to follow your finger or penlight with his or her eyes, without moving the head. You may hold the patient's chin gently with the other hand. Move your finger or penlight slowly up, down, left, and right. A routine check for convergence is not necessary, as it has little clinical value. EOMs can be assessed in an unconscious patient or in a patient suspected of having supranuclear palsy or ocular myopathy (fixed ophthalmoplegia) by testing oculocephalic (doll's eye) or oculovestibular reflexes (using the caloric test).

What to Note When Checking Extraocular Eye Movements

- At rest both eyes are aligned or deviated (conjugated or dysconjugated)
- Spontaneous eye movements (nystagmus)
- One or more CNs are affected
- Complaints of diplopia
- Any pupillary abnormalities or ptosis
- Any focal neurologic deficits

Eye Movement Abnormalities

Eye movement abnormalities may arise in the following situations:

- From a lesion affecting supranuclear gaze centers, which include frontal lobes, occipital lobes, and cerebellovestibular pathway (e.g., stroke, progressive supranuclear palsy, Parkinson's disease)
- From a brain stem lesion affecting CN III, IV, or VI nuclei (e.g., stroke, brain stem glioma)
- From a brain stem lesion affecting internuclear connections of CN III, IV, or VI by involving the medial longitudinal fasciculus (known as **internuclear ophthalmoplegia**) (e.g., multiple sclerosis, stroke, brain stem glioma)
- From a lesion affecting CNs (e.g., compressive third nerve palsy, diabetic ophthalmoplegia, ophthalmoplegic migraine)
- From a neuromuscular disorder (e.g., ocular myasthenia gravis)

- From primary muscle disease (myotonic muscular dystrophy, oculopharyngeal muscular dystrophy, mitochondrial myopathies)

Caveat: Diplopia is the prime symptom of many acquired EOM disorders. Supranuclear and internuclear lesions and primary ocular myopathies usually do not manifest as diplopia.

Nystagmus

- Nystagmus is classified according to the direction of the fast component.
- A few beats of unsustained (transient) jerky eye movements on extreme horizontal gaze are not abnormal.
- Nystagmus can be caused by physiologic factors, an inner ear disorder (vestibulopathy), brain stem and cerebellar lesions, or retinal disease (inability to fixate).
- Isolated (without any associated neurologic signs) acquired vertical or horizontal nystagmus usually is drug induced, as from antiepileptic drug overdose.
- Horizontal nystagmus is common. Vertical nystagmus, if not drug induced, is caused by a brain stem or posterior fossa lesion.
- Vestibular (peripheral) nystagmus is differentiated from brain stem (central) nystagmus by being unsustained, fatigable, associated with vertigo and nausea, and reduced by fixation.
- Multidirectional nystagmus can be caused by drugs, alcohol, or a posterior fossa lesion.

- Dissociated or ataxic nystagmus manifests as a palsy of adduction of one eye and nystagmus of abducting the eye. This condition is often referred to as *internuclear ophthalmoplegia*; if this is seen in a young patient and is bilateral, multiple sclerosis should be suspected.
- When checking for nystagmus, hold your finger at about a 45-degree angle from the patient's eye. Slowly move your finger in four directions, then briefly pause it, as in a check for EOMs. The patient should be able to see your finger with both eyes.

Additional Extraocular Movement Abnormalities

- Lateral gaze palsy is commonly seen in hemispheric stroke. The patient looks away from the paralyzed side but toward site of lesion; it is correctable by the doll's eye maneuver or caloric reflex.
- Disconjugate gaze palsy is seen in brain stem (pontine) lesions; the eye does not move by doll's eye maneuver.
- Upward or downward gaze palsy is usually caused by a pontomesencephalic lesion.
- In supranuclear palsy (as seen in progressive supranuclear palsy and Parkinson's disease), the eyes move with the caloric test (by reflex induction, not voluntarily).
- Bilateral internuclear ophthalmoplegia can be caused by a medial longitudinal fasciculus lesion. In young

patients it can suggest multiple sclerosis or pontine glioma; in elderly patients it can indicate brain stem stroke.

Examination of the Face (Cranial Nerves V and VII)

The clinical presentation of abnormalities of CNs V and VII is facial numbness or a drooping face.

Cranial Nerve V (Trigeminal Nerve)

CN V is examined as follows:

- **Motor:** Feel the mastication muscles; feel the contraction of the masseter and temporalis muscles while the patient's teeth are clenched; and feel for resistance to jaw opening or closing.
- **Jaw jerk:** Ask the patient to open his or her mouth slightly, with the chin relaxed. With your finger placed gently on the patient's chin, tap your finger gently with a percussion hammer. Most normal individuals have no jaw jerk. Increased or brisk jaw jerk indicates upper motor neuron lesion with localization of the lesion above the foramen magnum.
- **Corneal reflex:** I recommend testing the corneal reflex (CR) in a patient with Bell's palsy, a comatose patient, or a patient suspected of having a brain stem or cavernous sinus lesion. The afferent limb of this reflex is supplied by CN V, and the efferent limb by CN VII.

Using a cotton ball (not a cotton swab or paper), touch the edge of the cornea while the patient looks in the opposite direction (left or right, up or down). Note any ipsilateral and contralateral eye blink. You also can check CR by blowing air on the eye (a technique particularly useful in comatose patients or patients unable to keep their eyes open). If the patient is conscious and aware, ask if the sensation of both corneal touch tests felt the same. Do not touch the cornea briskly, or you will induce a reflex blink response. Touch only the cornea, not the sclera, which does not respond to touch (a common mistake by students). The corneal reflex is decreased or absent in patients who wear contact lenses. When CR is absent bilaterally, consider a trigeminal nerve or pontine lesion; if it is absent unilaterally, consider a pontine or cerebellopontine lesion.

- **Sensory:** Sensation of the face controlled by branches V1, V2, and V3 of CN V. To test sensation, start by checking light touch first, then pinprick, so the patient accommodates to touch testing. In cases of sensory loss, try to determine branch distribution. If there is a defect in the light touch and pinprick reflexes, also check temperature. The trigeminal nerve does not control sensation at the jaw angle.
  - Sensory loss in the distribution of V1 may indicate herpes or cavernous sinus thrombosis.
  - Sensory loss in the distribution of V2 is suggestive of trauma.

- Sensory loss in the distribution of V3 may indicate basal tumor or meningitis.
- Sensory loss in the distribution of all branches of CN V indicates geniculate ganglion, sensory root, or nucleus lesion such as basilar meningitis or pontine lesion.
- Sensory loss of light touch only indicates sensory root lesion.
- Sensory loss of pain and temperature indicates brain stem lesion.
- Sensory loss in the distribution of V2 or V3 indicates possible carcinoma.
- Sensory loss around the mouth is suggestive of syringomyelia.

Cranial Nerve VII (Facial Nerve)

CN VII controls the following:

- Muscles of facial expression
- Tensor tympani and stapedius muscles
- Taste on the anterior two-thirds of the tongue
- Salivation and lacrimation

The sensory portion of the facial nerve supplies the external auditory canal up to the tragus of the ear.

Examination

1. Note any facial asymmetry between the nasolabial folds or forehead wrinkles.

2. As you look for asymmetry, ask the patient to show his or her teeth, whistle, or wrinkle the forehead.
3. Gently check resistance of eye closure muscles. Note any weakness of lower face and forehead muscles on the same side.
4. The sense of taste is not routinely tested. When a patient complains of lack of taste, check each side of the anterior two-thirds of the tongue and the posterior one-third separately with normal saline and sugar solutions.

Some Clinical Hints

- Slight facial asymmetry without facial weakness is insignificant; asymmetry that disappears on voluntary expression or smiling also is insignificant.
- A flat face in Parkinson's disease does not indicate bilateral facial nerve lesion.
- **Facial nerves pull down the eyelids and close the eyes; the third nerve, on the other hand, keeps the eyes open; therefore, ptosis is not caused by a facial nerve lesion.**

Interpretation

- Lower facial and forehead muscle weakness is consistent with **lower motor neuron** (LMN) weakness.
- An outward, upward rolling of the eyeball when the patient attempts to close his or her eyes is known as *Bell's phenomenon.*

- Isolated unilateral LMN facial weakness is seen in Bell's palsy.
- Bilateral LMN facial weakness is seen in sarcoidosis, Lyme neuropathy, and Guillain-Barré syndrome.
- Lower facial muscle weakness with relative preservation of the forehead muscles is consistent with **upper motor neuron** (UMN) weakness.
- UMN facial weakness plus ipsilateral, appendicular (limb) neurologic deficit indicates supratentorial lesion (as seen in stroke) and tumor.
- UMN facial weakness plus contralateral appendicular neurologic deficit indicates brain stem lesion.
- Bilateral UMN facial weakness associated with dysarthria, dysphagia, and inappropriate laughing and crying, indicates corticobulbar tract lesion, known as *pseudobulbar palsy*, and is often seen in bilateral strokes.

Examination of the Hearing and Vestibular Systems (Cranial Nerve VIII)

Hearing

Examination

Note if the patient appears to have hearing impairment or complains of hearing difficulty during normal conversation. Formal audiologic testing is mandatory in cases with hearing loss.

1. The ear canals should be checked for ear wax with an otoscope. The simplest, quickest way to check

hearing is to rub your fingers together in the front of each ear while masking the other ear.

2. If you find a hearing defect, proceed with the **Rinne test** and **Weber's test**.

   • The Rinne test compares bone conduction with air conduction. Hold a tuning fork (512–516 Hz) firmly over the patient's mastoid until the vibration sound disappears; then place the fork in front of the patient's ear. Normally, the patient should still hear the humming.

   • Weber's test is used to differentiate between hearing impairment of conducive or sensorineural origin. Place the stem of a vibrating tuning fork on the vertex or midline of the patient's forehead. If the sound is heard best in the affected ear, the impairment probably is conducive; if the sound is heard best in the normal ear, the impairment probably is sensorineural.

Interpretation

• In conductive hearing loss, bone conducive sound reception is better than air conducive sound reception. This commonly results from middle ear disease or accumulated ear wax.

• In sensorineural hearing loss, air conducive sound reception is better than bone conducive sound reception in one ear, but just the opposite in the other ear. This is seen in conditions such as Ménière's disease, meningitis, cerebellopontine lesions, or brain stem disease.

Examining the Vestibular System

1. Find out whether the patient experiences dizziness. This symptom could indicate vestibular disease.
2. When testing eye movements, note any nystagmus.
3. If the patient presents with acute vertigo, determine whether it is caused by inner ear disease (vestibulopathy) or a brain stem lesion. Use a head-tilt test, such as Nylen-Barany maneuver or Hallpike's test, to test for nystagmus and vertigo: While the patient sits on an examining table, check eye movement for nystagmus. Turn the patient's head left and right. Then have the patient lie down and hang his or her head from the table. In each position, check for nystagmus and vertigo. If the patient immediately develops vertigo and nystagmus, consider brain stem lesion. If vertigo and nystagmus develop after a delay and are fatigued, consider an inner ear disorder. If an inner ear disorder is suspected, proceed with the caloric test.

Caveat: The caloric test in a conscious patient is best performed in a laboratory because the patient may develop severe dizziness or nausea. To check for fast component or nystagmus in an awake patient, irrigate the ear with water at room temperature (not cold). In a normal ear, warm water produces a rotatory nystagmus on the side of stimulation. Cold irrigation causes a reaction on the side opposite of the stimulation.

Examination of the Mouth (Cranial Nerves IX, X, and XII)

CNs IX, X, and XII control the tongue, pharynx, and larynx.

Tongue

Examination

1. Inspect the patient's tongue in his or her mouth for atrophy and fasciculation.
2. Inspect the protruded tongue for tongue deviation.
3. Move the patient's protruded tongue from side to side, and note any asymmetry of movement.

Interpretation

- In an LMN lesion, the tongue deviates toward the side of the lesion; in UMN lesion, the tongue deviates away from the side of the lesion and is often associated with hemiparesis.
- Bilateral LMN lesions present with tongue weakness and often are associated with tongue atrophy and fasciculation.
- Bilateral UMN lesions present with tongue weakness and often are associated with hyperactive gag reflex and labile affect (pseudobulbar palsy).

Caveat: Small, tremorlike movements when the patient's tongue is protruded should not be mistaken for fasciculation. Fasciculation occurs when the tongue is resting in the mouth. In patients with unilateral facial muscle weakness, the tongue appears to be deviated. Do not mistake this for a CN XII lesion. Tongue deviation can be corrected by lifting the weak facial muscle.

Pharynx

Examination

1. Ask the patient to open his or her mouth. Note the position of the uvula spontaneously and by having the patient say "ah." Also note soft palate and uvula movement.
2. I test the gag reflex when a patient has dysarthria or dysphagia. To test the gag reflex, touch the pharyngeal wall with a cotton applicator, and note the symmetry of palate movements and movements of the uvula. Ask the patient to describe the sensation difference between the sides. The afferent arm of the gag reflex is CN IX; the efferent is CN X.

Interpretation

- If the uvula moves to one side, consider a CN X lesion.
- There is an absence of gag reflex palate movement in LMN lesion.
- Hyperactive gag reflex is seen in UMN lesions.

Larynx

Examination

1. Ask the patient to cough and drink a glass of water.

2. Consult an ear, nose, and throat specialist for direct vocal cord function, if necessary.

Interpretation

- Poor cough is usually seen in vocal cord palsy.
- Unilateral, recurrent laryngeal nerve palsy (vagus) presents with hoarseness and is commonly seen in middle-aged men.
- Dysphagia followed by cough (choking) is seen in tenth nerve palsy.
- Dysarthria, dysphagia, hoarseness, Horner's syndrome, and contralateral sensory loss with ipsilateral cerebellar dysfunction are indicative of brain stem lesion (lateral medullary syndrome).

Examination of the Shoulders and Neck (Cranial Nerve XI)

CN XI, the spinal accessory nerve, has branches from the medulla and cervical spinal roots of C2–C4 and innervates the sternocleidomastoid and the trapezius muscles.

Examination

1. Examine the neck and shoulders for wasting and fasciculation of the sternocleidomastoid and trapezius muscles and for shoulderdrop.
2. Ask the patient to shrug his or her shoulders. Check the resistance as you push down, and note asymmetry. To check the sternocleidomastoid muscle, ask the patient to resist against your push to the right

and left jaw angle (temporomandibular joint). Note the strength and bulk of the sternocleidomastoid muscles and any asymmetry.

Interpretation

- Ipsilateral weakness of the trapezius and sternocleido-mastoid muscles indicates peripheral eleventh nerve palsy. If this is associated with ninth and tenth nerve palsy, consider foramen jugular lesion.
- Weakness of the sternocleidomastoid on one side and trapezius on the other side is seen in ipsilateral UMN lesion.
- Unilateral inability to shrug is caused by contralateral UMN lesion.
- Bilateral weakness and atrophy of sternocleidomastoid muscles usually are seen in myotonic muscular dystrophy, fascioscapulohumeral muscular dystrophy or motor neuron disease.
- Ipsilateral weakness of the trapezius (inability to shrug) and hemiparesis suggests internal capsule infarction in the distribution of the anterior cerebral artery.
- Unilateral sternomastoid weakness is rare, and usually is post-traumatic.

SENSORY EXAMINATION

Anatomy

Pain and temperature sensations travel through the spinothalamic tract and cross at the spinal cord level; proprioceptive sensation travels through the posterior column and crosses at the medulla. Higher cortical sensation is the primary function of the parietal lobes.

Examination

Sensory screening includes

- Vibration, joint position sense, light touch (proprioceptive)
- Pain and temperature (exteroceptive)
- Stereognosis, graphesthesia, two-point discrimination, double-simultaneous stimulation (higher cortical sensory)

The sensory system should be screened in all patients. During the screening, which must be done in an organized manner, concentration and patience are required by both the examiner and patient. Explain to the patient what you are doing and demonstrate it. Tell the patient the type of response you expect.

1. Start the sensory testing with screenings for light touch, vibration, and joint position because these are less stressful to the patient and allow you to assess the patient's reliability.
2. Ensure you are comparing the sensory function between left and right and distal and proximal.
3. Start the sensory testing with the problem area, then move to a normal area. Sensory examination is complementary to the motor system. Sensory test-

ing helps establish whether the deficit is in the distribution of one nerve, multiple nerves, or root; whether the sensory deficit is symmetric, asymmetric, or distal versus proximal; and, most important, whether the deficit is segmental (level). Often the patient has mapped the sensory deficit in the history and description of the problem. Your job is to confirm or dispute the sensory loss.

Testing for Light Touch

Ask the patient to say "yes" when an area of the body is touched. Then, using a small piece of cotton, dab (do not rub) the patient's skin while the patient's eyes are closed. Pause a few seconds between each touch. Quantitate the test by comparing touch and nontouch, thus mapping the area of abnormality.

Testing for Vibration

When testing for vibration, explain to the patient that you will be using a tuning fork. Demonstrate by touching the vibrating tuning fork to the patient's chin or forehead. Ask the patient to report buzzing or humming, but not a sense of touch. While the patient's eyes are closed, place a vibrating 128-Hz tuning fork on a bony prominence. Start distally (dorsum of the toes) and move proximally. If the distal area is normal, you do not need to move proximally. Determine the patient's threshold for perceiving low-intensity vibration. Ask the patient to report when he or she no longer feels vibration; compare the patient's perceptions with your own. Vibration can be objectively tested by comparing the patient's ability to feel buzzing and touching.

Testing for Joint Position Sense

Joint position sense and proprioception can be tested several ways:

- **Moving toes or fingers up and down:** With the patient's eyes open, demonstrate how you will move his or her toes or fingers up and down. Ask the patient to close his or her eyes. Hold the big toe on the sides. With the other hand, stabilize the joint, then make large movements, decreasing to smaller and smaller movements until the patient makes an error in perception. The fourth toe is the most sensitive for detecting subtle joint position sense deficit. The test can be objective by assessing the degree of joint movements. If joint movements are not possible or are difficult to assess, an easy test is to ask the patient, eyes open or closed, to extend his or her arms to the side, then bring the index fingers of both hands together.

- **Romberg's test:** Romberg's test assesses the posterior column function and is easier to do while testing station and gait. Ask the patient to stand, feet together, with arms in front of the face, eyes closed. If the patient begins to fall when the eyes are closed, the Romberg's test is positive.

Remember: Stand beside or behind the patient so that you can catch the patient if necessary. This test cannot be performed if the patient is unable to stand without assistance.

- **Directional scratch test:** Instead of standard vibration and joint position testing, the easiest way to check posterior column function is by directional scratch test. With the tip of a blunt object (e.g., tongue blade) randomly stroke a 2-cm long scratch over palm and midsole and ask the patient to tell you the direction of the scratch.

Pinprick Test

Begin the pinprick test by explaining and demonstrating the test to the patient (sharp versus dull, symmetry). Using a safety pin, establish the patient's threshold to the least intensity of stimulus. Begin distally in an abnormal area and move proximally toward a normal area to map the sensory loss.

Testing for Temperature Sensitivity

Testing for temperature sensitivity is not routine. Most neurologists check temperature sensation when the patient reports an abnormality or a specific disease indicates it (e.g., syringomyelia). An informal check can be done by touching the patient's skin with the cold metal of a percussion hammer, then the warmer rubber head of the hammer. Formal temperature testing is done using a tube of cold water (dry the exterior of the tube first) and a tube of warm water. **Some neurologists, however, prefer the temperature test instead of pinprick because it is painless and provides nearly the same information.**

Double-Simultaneous Stimulation

Begin double-simultaneous stimulation by demonstrating what you are going to do and what type of response is expected. Ask the patient to close his or her eyes as you randomly touch different parts of the body with a cotton ball or the tip of your finger. Touch either one spot at a time or two different spots simultaneously. Abnormal double-simultaneous stimulation suggests a nondominant parietal lobe lesion.

Some Clinical Hints

- Memorize sensory deficits in the distribution of median, ulnar, radial, and axillary nerves in the upper extremity and lateral femoral cutaneous, femoral, sciatic and peroneal nerves in the lower extremities.
- Memorize the common segmental sensory levels: shoulder pad (C4), nipple (T4), umbilicus (T10), and groin (L1).
- A sensory deficit can be seen in any lesion affecting a single peripheral nerve to the parietal lobe and even psychogenic (hyperventilation). To locate the problem, combine the sensory abnormalities with the other neurologic findings.

MOTOR SYSTEM EXAMINATION

Strength, Muscle Tone, Bulk, Reflexes

- When examining a patient complaining of weakness, establish the following:
  - Muscles are weak objectively or just fatigued
  - Onset, course, and distribution of weakness
  - Cause of weakness (e.g., due to UMN, LMN lesion, or nonorganic [functional])
- LMN weakness is characterized by normal or decreased muscle tone, hyporeflexia or areflexia, atrophy, and fasciculation with or without sensory deficit.
- UMN weakness is characterized by weakness of extensor muscles in the upper extremities and flexors in the lower extremities; hypotonia or hypertonia, hyperreflexia, clonus, and the presence of pathologic reflexes.
- Functional weakness is characterized by nonanatomic, erratic (give-away) weakness; discrepancy between voluntary use of muscles by the patient; and, when tested directly, normal reflexes, tone, and sensory examination.
- The following Medical Research Council scale commonly is used to demonstrate the degree of weakness by manual muscle testing.

Normal	5
Moderate movement against resistance	4
Mild movement against resistance	3
Movement when gravity is eliminated	2

Trace of movement	1
No movement	0

- **Caveat:** Limb pain caused by soft tissue, bone, or joint disease and limb position affect strength testing.
- **Caveat:** Test the muscle when the limb is in midposition, neither completely flexed nor extended (locked position).
- Muscle weakness should be interpreted in the context of muscle tone, bulk, and reflexes, as well as other associated neurologic signs.

Muscle Tone

Tone is increased resistance by passive movements of the limb at the joint level. Tone examination often is neglected because the patient does not complain of a tone problem. Tone in upper extremities is checked at the wrist and elbow joints; it is checked in the lower extremities at the knee level. Ask the patient to relax the joint, then check the tone.

Tone is measured in three levels:

1. Normal
2. Decreased
   a. Hypotonia (mild)
   b. Flaccid (severe)
3. Increased
   a. **Spasticity**, increased tone throughout range of motion followed by a sudden release (catch), as seen in a UMN lesion.

b. **Rigidity**, increased tone throughout the range of motion, is called cogwheel rigidity if is intermittent and ratchet-like. Cogwheel rigidity is seen in extrapyramidal diseases such as Parkinson's disease.

c. **Paratonia**, or **gegenhalten**, which is increased tone, appears when the patient opposes the movement of a limb. It is seen in a bifrontal lobe lesion and diffuse encephalopathy.

d. **Myotonia**, delay in muscle relaxation after the muscle is activated, either spontaneously (e.g., handgrip myotonia) or induced by percussion (e.g., percussion myotonia), is typically seen in myotonic muscular dystrophy.

e. **Dystonia**, contraction of agonist and antagonist muscle, producing sustained abnormal limb posture, is seen in extrapyramidal disorders.

Muscle Atrophy and Fasciculation

Muscle atrophy and fasciculation (twitching of muscle fascicle) commonly are seen in an LMN lesion such as in motor neuron diseases, radiculopathy, or chronic polyneuropathies. Consider muscular dystrophy when there is generalized muscle wasting without fasciculations. Disuse atrophy is seen after stroke or when a limb is casted.

Caveat: Fasciculations without muscle atrophy, weakness, or reflex changes can indicate benign (physiologic) or drug-induced (cholinergics) reactions. Fasciculation is difficult to detect in obese individuals and newborns (check hands, pectoralis, or tongue muscles). Hands in elderly patients (senile hands) may appear to have intrinsic muscle wasting, but strength (grip) is good when tested.

Clinical Observations

Subtle unilateral weakness caused by a UMN lesion can be detected by the following tests:

- **Pronator sign:** Ask the patient to extend his or her arms in front, palms up, fingers open, and close his or her eyes. Drifting of the arms with pronation of the hand indicates weakness caused by UMN.
- **Strength of wrist extensors:** Weakness of these muscles is seen early in the course of a UMN lesion.
- **Finger tapping:** Ask the patient to rapidly tap the fingers together; slowness or clumsiness indicates early UMN lesion; however, this sign should be interpreted within the context of the clinical history.
- **Foot circling sign:** This test checks for subtle weakness of distal lower extremity caused by UMN lesion. The sign is positive when the patient is unable or does a clumsy job when asked to circle his or her foot.
- **Forearm rolling:** The affected forearm cannot roll smoothly around the other.

Reflexes

There are four groups of reflexes: muscle stretch, superficial, corticobulbar, and pathologic.

General Rules When Testing Reflexes

- The preferred position for testing most reflexes is seated; however, abdominal, cremasteric, and Babinski's reflexes are best tested in the supine position.
- Feel the tendon for localization or tenderness and relax the patient's joint before tapping.
- Swing the hammer head to tap, do not just touch the tendon. The speed of the hammer head is important.
- A normal response to tapping may be a limb jerk, corresponding muscle twitch, or tendon twitch under your finger.
- Listen for the sound of the taps; true absence of reflexes sounds dull.
- Always check reflexes simultaneously between two sides to establish symmetry.
- Hypo- or hyperreflexia, if asymmetric, is clinically significant when associated with other neurologic signs.
- Bilateral absence of brachioradialis or ankle jerks in an asymptomatic patient is insignificant.
- Unilateral absence of ankle jerks is consistent with an S1 root lesion.
- Do reinforcement before concluding a reflex is absent.

- Asymmetry of reflexes is significant when it is reproducible.
- Ankle jerks commonly are absent in patients 60 years and older; therefore, there is no need to check ankle jerks in these patients.

Superficial Reflexes

Superficial reflexes are elicited by stroking the skin (e.g., abdominal, cremasteric, plantar) or mucous membranes (e.g., gag, corneal). The **plantar** response is the most important superficial reflex and should be checked in all patients with neurologic presentations. Most superficial reflexes are polysynaptic and are affected by a segmental (root, nerve) lesion, as well as suprasegmental (cortical, brain stem) lesions.

OBTAINING THE PLANTAR RESPONSE

The plantar response is best obtained when the patient is supine. Explain the procedure to the patient. With one hand, hold the patient's ankle. With the other hand, using a blunt object such as a key or broken tongue blade, stroke from the lateral border of the foot across to the foot pad. Observe for the following responses:

- All toes flex (flexor plantar response): normal
- Big toe extends and other toes spread (extensor plantar response or Babinski's): abnormal
- Only big toe extends (toe sign, up-going toe): abnormal

- Foot dorsiflexes, knee flexes, and hip flexes (triple flexor response): abnormal
- Foot and knee show nonstereotypical flexion (withdraw response): normal
- No movement: no response

INTERPRETATION

- Flexor plantar response is normal.
- No response is seen in some normal individuals or patients with severe weakness or neuropathy.
- Nonstereotypical flexor response is withdrawal.
- Babinski's sign, extensor toe sign, and stereotypical triple flexor response are abnormal and indicate UMN lesion involving pyramidal tract from the L2 spinal cord level to the cerebral cortex.

Caveat: The withdrawal response can be reduced in some sensitive (ticklish) patients. By repeating the plantar reflex, some patients adapt. Use less pressure and stroke the lateral aspect of the sole without crossing the foot pad and note big toe movement. If you are unsuccessful, use an alternate stimuli (e.g., stroke the lateral aspect of the foot or Chaddock's sign, or gently prick the dorsum of the big toe [Bing sign]).

Caveat: The absence of Babinski's sign does not rule out UMN lesion, particularly in the acute stage (stroke). The presence of Babinski's sign without any other UMN sign should be interpreted with caution.

Corticobulbar Reflexes

The jaw jerk and snout reflexes are mediated through the corticobulbar tract. They are clinically significant when they are hyperactive, indicating bilateral UMN lesions. For example, in patients with a suspected UMN lesion, a brisk jaw jerk indicates the lesion is above the foramen magnum, most probably at or above the pontine level.

Remember: Tapping the chin or mouth too hard disturbs the patient and may produce a false-positive hyperactive response. To check the jaw jerk and the snout reflexes, place your left index finger on the patient's chin and mouth and tap gently.

Pathologic Reflexes

Pathologic reflexes commonly are known as the *frontal release signs* (i.e., grasp, glabellar, or palmomental). These signs are primitive; their presence indicates bifrontal lobe lesions or a diffuse CNS insult. The Hoffmann's or Tromner's reflex is elicited in some normal individuals, but asymmetric responses may be significant. A positive glabellar reflex (Meyerson's), which is induced by gently tapping (hammer or finger) the glabellar nerve, is commonly seen in Parkinson's disease. The reflex is positive when the patient continues to blink each time the nerve is tapped.

Gait

Gait should be tested in all patients when possible because it is a function of the motor, sensory, and cerebellar systems. It is unlikely a patient with serious neurologic problems will have a normal gait. Adequate gait testing requires approximately 20 feet of walking space. Testing the patient while he or she is barefoot is best. You should be able to see the patient's arms and legs (have the patient dress in a hospital gown or underwear or roll the pants up to the knees). Be prepared to protect the patient from a fall, particularly with hemiparetic, ataxic, or elderly patients.

Examination

1. Ask the patient to walk as usual. Note whether the gait is broad-based, symmetric or asymmetric, or the arms swing.
2. After the patient has demonstrated the gait, ask the patient to walk on his or her toes, heels, and heel-to-toe.
3. You may want to examine the patient for Romberg's sign when checking gait.

Examples of Abnormal Gaits

- Difficulty initiating walk (**gait apraxia**) can indicate normal pressure hydrocephalus.
- Broad-based, uncoordinated gait with staggering (**ataxia**) can indicate cerebellar disease.

- Short-stepped gait with stooped posture and little or no arm swing can indicate Parkinson's disease or drug-induced parkinsonism.
- Short-stepped gait with erect posture and arm swing (**marche à petits pas**) can indicate diffuse cerebrovascular disease.
- Legs crossed over (**scissoring**) can indicate bilateral UMN lesions or cerebral palsy.
- Marked pelvic and shoulder rotation (**waddling**) can indicate myopathy or muscular dystrophy.
- Bizarre, inconsistent, and worse-when-watched gait (**functional**) can indicate a psychogenic condition.
- Painful, limping (**antalgic**) gait can indicate acute lumbar disk herniation.
- One leg swinging out and adducting (**circumduction**) can indicate hemiparesis caused by UMN lesion.
- High knee lift on one side accompanied by feet slapping down (**steppage**) can indicate footdrop (peroneal palsy) or L5 root lesion.
- Non-neurologic gait difficulties include arthritis and orthopedic problems.

Coordination and Cerebellar Function Tests

Upper Extremity

Upper extremity coordination and cerebellar function tests include the following:

- **Finger-to-nose test:** This test is best done with the patient in a sitting position. Stay in front of the patient, and hold your index finger about an arm's length from the patient. Ask the patient to touch your finger with his or her index finger, then the tip of his or her nose. Make sure the patient's arm is extended. You may move your target finger in different directions. The task is to be done slowly, then faster. Check one arm at a time. If the patient develops a tremor when approaching the target (intention tremor), cerebellar disease should be suspected. The patient's missing the target indicates past-pointing or **dysmetria**.

- **Rapid alternating movements:** Ask the patient to demonstrate finger tapping or hand tapping, first in slow motion, then faster. Check one hand at a time. Doing the task with regular rate and rhythm is normal. Irregular, disorganized, or dysrhythmic movements indicate incoordination (**dysdiadochokinesia**), suggestive of cerebellar disease.

- **Rebound test:** To protect the patient's face and eyes, place a hand on the patient's shoulder and ask him or her to turn the head in the opposite direction. Then ask the patient to flex the opposite elbow and resist as you try to extend his or her arm. Suddenly let the arm go. Check one side at a time. The results are normal if the arm returns to steadying position. Positive rebound is when the arm oscillates several times then stays.

- **Alternate rebound test:** Ask the patient to straighten his or her arm in the air and resist as you push it down, then let the arm go. The reaction is abnormal if the arms bounce before they stop.

Lower Extremity

Lower extremity coordination and cerebellar function tests include the following:

- **Heel-to-toe testing:** Check when testing gait. Approximately 20 feet of walking space is required. Ask the patient to walk heel-to-toe in a straight line. The results are abnormal (**ataxia**) if the patient falls to one side or becomes unsteady.
- **Heel-to-shin testing:** Best results are achieved with the patient supine. Ask the patient to lift one leg and place his or her heel on the shin of the other leg, then smoothly rub it down toward the toes. The result is abnormal if the movement is irregular or if the heel falls off the leg. Make sure the patient rubs his or her heel, not foot pad, on the shin. Repeat the test several times, if necessary.
- **Foot or heel tapping testing:** This test is similar to rapid alternating movements test in the upper extremity.

Trunk

Trunk coordination and cerebellar functions are tested in the following way: Ask the patient to sit up from a supine position without using his or her hands. If the patient falls to one side, **truncal ataxia** is indicated. Ask the patient to stand on his or her feet. If the patient becomes unsteady and has a tendency to fall, again, **truncal ataxia** is indicated. The patient's eyes remain open in both tests.

Clinical Considerations

- Unilateral or bilateral limb ataxia or incoordination is seen in a cerebellar hemisphere lesion.
- Truncal ataxia indicates midline or superior vermis pathology.
- Other signs of cerebellar dysfunction include nystagmus, tremor, dysarthric speech and, less frequently, hypotonia and pendular reflexes.

Caveats: Severe loss of joint position sense can produce incoordination (sensory ataxia). The difference between cerebellar ataxia and sensory ataxia is that sensory ataxia is worse when the eyes are closed. In sensory ataxia, the outstretched hand (when the eyes are closed) may show abnormal incoordinated movement (pseudoathetosis).

Caveats

- A patient with motor weakness on one side (e.g., stroke) may show clumsiness in finger-to-nose or heel-to-shin testing. This weakness is not caused by a cerebellar disorder; the movement is slow but not irregular. Coordination can be corrected by holding the weak limb and then asking the patient to do the task.

- Patients with Parkinson's disease or essential tremor may perform finger-to-nose testing poorly because of rigidity and tremor.
- A normal finger-to-nose test does not rule out a cerebellar lesion because, in a midline cerebellar lesion, this task can be preserved.

2

Neurologic Formulation

A neurologic formulation is a summary of findings from a patient's history and examination. It should include information about the following:

- Probable anatomic site
- Probable etiology
- Differential diagnosis
- Diagnostic tests to support hypothesis or exclude possibilities
- Therapeutic plan, counseling, and referral

Formulation is based on neurologic history and findings, but it may be necessary to reformulate as laboratory data become available or as the patient's problem evolves.

MODIFIED NEUROLOGIC EXAMINATION

Examination of a new patient usually begins by addressing the chief complaint, followed by a complete examination (e.g., in a patient with back pain radiating to the leg, you may start by examining the back and lower extremities, then explore other areas). A **focused examination** usually is performed when a patient returns for a follow-up visit, unless the neurologic history suggests a recent change.

Generally, an effort should made to complete both a thorough neurologic history and examination; however, in some cases, such as with comatose patients, pediatric patients, and agitated, uncooperative patients, it is not possible to do so. Such patients may require a limited neurologic history and examination. Sometimes, in an agitated or uncooperative patient, careful observation of the patient's behavior can replace a more formal examination.

3

Neurologic Signs of Interest

MARCUS GUNN PUPIL

Marcus Gunn pupil (relative afferent pupillary defect) is a unilateral paradoxic dilation in one eye when a direct light beam is oscillated between a patient's eyes. It is seen in an optic nerve lesion anterior to the optic chiasm, such as retrobulbar optic neuritis or optic neuritis (papillitis); it is also seen in compressive optic nerve lesions or retinal degeneration.

LHERMITTE'S SIGN

Lhermitte's sign (barber's chair sign) is a sensation of electrical shock or paresthesia running down the back when the neck is flexed or extended. This sign usually is seen in a cervical cord lesion such as demyelinating disease (multiple sclerosis), cervical spondylotic myelopathy, or cervical spinal cord tumor.

BRUDZINSKI'S AND KERNIG'S SIGNS

Brudzinski's and Kernig's signs are best detected when the patient lies flat. Brudzinski's sign occurs during passive flexion of the neck, resulting in flexion of the knees and hips. Kernig's sign is demonstrated as resistance to straightening a flexed knee. These signs indicate meningeal irritation (e.g., meningitis, subarachnoid hemorrhage), and they are not evident when neck stiffness is not caused by meningeal irritation, such as in cervical spondylosis, parkinsonism, or cervical lymphadenopathy. Unilateral Kernig's sign may be seen in lumbar radiculopathy.

TINEL'S SIGN

Tinel's sign is paresthesias in the distribution of the sensory branches of the median nerve elicited by a gentle percussion applied at the distal end of a limb. This sign is often elicited in carpal tunnel syndrome and other entrapment neuropathies (e.g., cubital tunnel syndrome).

FROMENT'S PAPER SIGN

Froment's paper sign, flexion of the distal phalanx of the thumb elicited when a piece of paper is pulled between the thumb and index finger, is a result of a weak adductor pollicis; the long flexor compensates. Froment's sign indicates a lesion of the ulnar nerve at the elbow, either unilateral or bilateral.

STRAIGHT LEG RAISING TEST

With the patient in a supine position, lift the leg while holding the heel. Limitation of leg raise to 45–60 degrees suggests nerve root compression. Hamstring muscle tightness does not indicate radiculopathy.

PATRICK'S TEST

With the patient supine, the heel on the symptomatic side is placed on the opposite knee and passive pressure is applied on the leg down and out. If pain occurs in the hip, sacroiliac joint disease is indicated.

PRONATION SIGN

The pronation sign appears as pronation of the forearm caused by passive flexion. It is seen in hemiplegia. With eyes closed, the patient extends his or her hands, palms up. A drift of the arm with pronation of the hand indicates motor weakness caused by upper motor neuron lesion.

HOOVER'S SIGN

When a patient with hemiparesis attempts to raise the weak leg, excessive downward pressure can be felt on the examiner's hand placed under the heel of the normal leg. In hysterical weakness, the lack of downward pressure on the normal leg suggests that no effort is being made to elevate the affected one (positive Hoover's).

TODD'S PARALYSIS

Todd's paralysis, often mistaken for stroke or transient ischemic attack, is a transient hemiparesis after focal motor seizure (postictal weakness).

HALLPIKE'S TEST

Hallpike's test, or the head-tilt test, is used to evaluate positional vertigo (see Chapter 1). The patient's head, gently supported, hangs off the bed while the examiner moves the head right and left. Normally, there is no nystagmus. With inner ear disease, the patient develops vertigo and nystagmus, which is fatigable, after a few seconds. When a central lesion is present, nystagmus occurs without delay and does not fatigue.

PUPILLARY SPARING

Pupillary sparing is retention of pupillary reaction to light in cases of third nerve palsy (ptosis and eye movement abnormalities). It is seen more often in ischemic third nerve palsy, such as in diabetics and hypertensive patients, and less frequently in compressive third nerve palsies, such as aneurysm or tumors.

FISHER'S SIGN

Fisher's sign appears when the middle joint of the thumb is tapped repeatedly with the tip of the index finger and the other fingers move synchronously. The absence of other finger movement indicates corticospinal tract lesion.

FOREARM-ROLLING SIGN

The forearm-rolling test involves rapidly rolling one arm around the other. In a subtle pyramidal tract lesion, one arm does not roll smoothly around the other.

4

Approach to the Patient with Suspected Hysteric Conversion

Neurologic symptoms (complaints) and signs (deficits) that are nonorganic and result from psychological factors are commonly encountered in neurologic practice.

WHEN TO SUSPECT HYSTERIC CONVERSION

Key indicators of hysteric conversion include the following:

- Motor or sensory symptoms not accompanied by objective deficit (e.g., reflex changes, muscle tone, atrophy)
- Nonanatomic motor or sensory deficit
- Patient unconcerned about deficits
- Possible secondary gain as motive
- Patient history of personality disorder or multiple hospitalizations

Hysteric conversion is difficult to diagnose. Moreover, it can be a convenient diagnosis in the absence of a clear-cut neurologic diagnosis. Some factors to weigh before offering a diagnosis of hysteric conversion include the following:

- Bizarre, purely subjective complaints neither exclude an organic lesion nor support a psychogenic (functional) disorder. For example, multiple sclerosis can present with bizarre, subjective, and multifocal (nonanatomic) symptoms.
- Eliminating neurologic disease as a diagnosis is important; however, the absence of neurologic disease does not indicate hysteric conversion as a diagnosis. The diagnosis should not only be based on exclusion of organic disorder but also supported by **positive signs** of conversion.
- Ordering extensive, expensive, invasive tests, surgical procedures, or drug therapy is inadvisable in suspected hysteric conversion.
- Examining a patient with suspected hysteria calls for special care to avoid embarrassment or feelings of threat.
- Concluding a diagnosis of hysteric conversion based on patient history and examination does not preclude the presence of a superimposed organic neurologic problem.

Because hysteric conversion is nonspecific, diagnosis is difficult. It is easy to make a premature diagnosis of hysteria. Sometimes a patient's behavior and personality can lead a practitioner to an incorrect diagnosis of hysteric conversion. Inconsistent patient responses during the sensory examination, which is subjective for both patient and examiner, can give a false impression. Likewise, some neurologic diseases (e.g., multiple sclerosis, transient ischemic attacks, small strokes, seizures, sleep and movement disorders, myasthenia gravis) are commonly mistaken as hysteria. **Numerous cases of misdiagnosed hysteria later are revealed as multiple sclerosis by magnetic resonance imaging.**

COMMON POSITIVE NEUROLOGIC SIGNS OF HYSTERIC CONVERSION

- **Memory loss:** All cognitive function tests are normal, except memory.
- **Unconsciousness:** When the patient's arms are held up, then suddenly dropped, the arms do not strike the patient's face; eyelids may show resistance to opening.
- **Blindness:** The eye examination is normal (i.e., pupils, visual field, discs, optokinetic nystagmus).
- **Deafness:** The patient responds to loud noise or music.
- **Anosmia:** The patient has no reaction to ammonia and alcohol (these substances irritate the trigeminal nerve in the mucosa and not the olfactory nerve).
- **Gait:** The patient exhibits staggering and reeling (astasia-abasia) but does not fall, holding the rail, furniture, wall, or examiner to prevent the fall and self-injury.
- **Sensory deficit:** The patient exhibits inconsistent, patchy sensory loss, ipsilateral sensory loss (vision, hearing, smell), or midline sensory deficits (splitting the midline). A tuning fork placed on the forehead,

chin, or sternal bone creates lateralized vibration. When a patient with hysteric conversion is touched during the touch test and asked to say "yes" when touched, he or she responds "yes" whether touched or not.

- **Weakness:** The patient exhibits maximum strength briefly, then irregular or give-away weakness. The patient's strength often improves with encouragement. The patient may contract the antagonist muscle instead. There may be no significant asymmetry of strength when arms checked simultaneously. Hoover's sign may be positive in lower extremity weakness

Hint: Indirectly testing patients (observing patients when they believe they are not being tested or misdirecting the patient's attention [e.g., checking strength while you discuss an unrelated subject]) may produce better results. Observe patients' activity during casual conversation.

5

Neuroanatomy of Localization

Localization, the determination of the site or place of a lesion, requires a basic, but not detailed, knowledge of neuroanatomy.

WHAT YOU SHOULD KNOW

- Blood supply and circulation of the cerebral cortex, internal capsule, basal ganglia, cerebellum, and brain stem (carotids and vertebrobasilar system)
- Function of cerebral cortex lobes (left and right)
- Internal capsule anatomy
- Brain stem nuclei and tracts
- Eye movement control system
- Pupillary control system
- Visual field pathway
- Autonomic bladder control
- Common root innervation of cervical, lumbosacral, and sacral spinal cord

OTHER IMPORTANT NEUROANATOMIC STRUCTURES

Long Tracts

Long tracts are prime structures of clinical neurology. These tracts cross; therefore, they lateralize neurologic symptoms and signs. Long tracts include the following:

- The **corticospinal tract (descending)** connects the cerebral cortex (precentral gyrus) to the spinal cord (lateral and ventral), passes through the anterior third of the internal capsule, and crosses at the lower medulla.
- The **corticobulbar tract (descending)** connects the cerebral cortex (precentral gyrus) to the brain stem nuclei (it crosses before connection to nuclei) and passes through the genu of internal capsule.
- The **spinothalamic tract (ascending)** connects skin (conducting pain and temperature) to the cerebral cortex (postcentral gyrus) on the contralateral side by synapsing to the third-order neuron, ventralis posterolateralis nucleus of the thalamus. This tract passes through the internal capsule posterior limb.
- The **dorsal column (lemniscal) tract (ascending)** connects skin, joint, and tendon sensation (proprioception) to the contralateral cerebral cortex (postcentral gyrus). It travels through the posterior limb of the internal capsule and synapses in the thalamus ventralis posterolateralis before ending in the cortex.

- The **visual tract (straight)** connects the retina to the occipital lobe and crosses at the optic chiasm.

The **medial longitudinal fasciculus** connects the nuclei of cranial nerves III, IV, and VI. It functions as efferent to the lateral vestibular nuclei, descends to the spinal cord, and is important in lateral eye movement.

Common Sensory Dermatomes

A dermatome is an area of skin supplied with afferent nerve fibers by a single posterior spinal root. **Common dermatomes** and their supplying nerves include the following:

Shoulder pad	C4
Thumb	C6
Little finger	C8
Nipple	T4
Umbilicus	T10
Groin	L1
Big toe	L5

6

Common Neurologic Constructs

SUBCORTICAL LESION (POSTERIOR LIMB, INTERNAL CAPSULE) VERSUS PARIETO-OCCIPITAL LOBE LESION

In subcortical lesion, motor weakness (paresis) usually affects the face, arm, and leg equally. The primary sensory deficits—paresthesia, numbness—are more prominent because the posterior limb of the internal capsule is involved. Cortical lesions affect higher cortical sensory function, manifesting as agnosia, agraphesthesia, and impairment of two-point discrimination.

Visual field defects are more common because visual tracts travel through the posterior limb of the internal capsule. Occipital lobe lesions produce visual field defects but usually are not associated with motor or sensory deficit. Dominant cortical lesion produces aphasia and apraxia.

GERSTMANN'S SYNDROME

Gerstmann's syndrome is commonly caused by stroke affecting the left angular and supramarginal gyri and is clinically characterized by finger agnosia, left-right disorientation, agraphia, and dyscalculia.

WATERSHED INFARCTS (BORDERZONE INFARCTS)

Watershed areas are end-artery zones between superficial branches of a major cortical blood supply (e.g., between the anterior cerebral artery and middle cerebral artery; between the middle cerebral artery and posterior cerebral artery). Bilateral watershed infarcts occur in severe hypotension or hypoxia; unilateral watershed infarcts occur when the affected artery is stenotic and collateral circulation cannot compensate in a hypotensive episode.

INTERNUCLEAR OPHTHALMOPLEGIA

Internuclear ophthalmoplegia (INO) is characterized by weakness of the adducting eye (site of lesion) and monocular nystagmus (dissociated nystagmus) of the abducting eye. Although INO can be seen in many brain stem lesions, bilateral INO (medial longitudinal fasciculus lesion) in young adults is most consistent with multiple sclerosis; in elderly individuals, it is caused by ischemic brain stem insults. Patients with INO usually do not complain of blurred or double vision.

WALLENBERG'S SYNDROME (LATERAL MEDULLARY SYNDROME)

Wallenberg's syndrome is caused by infarction of the medulla and cerebellum due to vertebral or posterior inferior cerebellar artery occlusion. It is characterized by the following:

- Ipsilaterally (to the site of the lesion) decreased pain and facial temperature
- Dysarthria; dysphagia; and ipsilateral decrease of palatal, pharyngeal, and vocal cord movements
- Ipsilateral Horner's syndrome
- Ipsilateral dystaxia
- Hiccup, vertigo, and nausea
- Contralateral body sensory loss (pain and temperature)

SPASTIC PARAPARESIS

Spastic paraparesis can be caused by the following:

- Spinal cord or brain stem lesion
- Hemispheric lesion
  - Bilateral frontal lobe infarction (occlusion of bilateral anterior cerebral arteries or watershed infarcts)
  - Hydrocephalus
  - Parasagittal mass (falx meningioma)
  - Callosal lesion

HALLMARKS OF BRAIN STEM LESIONS

Hallmarks of brain stem lesions include the following:

- Cranial nerve (CN) dysfunction
- Contralateral body motor and sensory deficits (crossed deficits)
- Cerebellar signs
- Gaze palsy
- Nystagmus
- Dysarthria
- Alteration of mental status and coma at onset of acute severe brain stem lesion

EXTRA-AXIAL BRAIN STEM LESION

Suspect an extra-axial lesion (without compressing brain stem) when multiple CN dysfunction is not associated with motor sensory deficit or altered mental status. Acoustic neuroma, meningioma, epidermoid cyst, and aneurysm are some causes.

PSEUDOBULBAR PALSY

In pseudobulbar palsy, lesions involving bilateral cortico-bulbar tracts manifest as dysarthria, dysphagia, drooling, and a labile effect (inappropriate laugh or cry). The bulbar muscles are weak but not atrophied.

CLUMSY HAND SYNDROME

Characterized by dysarthria, dysphagia, hand clumsiness, and often extensor plantar response (Babinski's sign), clumsy hand syndrome is commonly caused by a lacunar infarction in the base of the pons and sometimes the internal capsule.

HALLMARKS OF SPINAL CORD LESIONS

Hallmarks of spinal cord lesions include the following:

- Sensory level deficit
- Bilateral extremity weakness, with distal greater than proximal
- Bowel or bladder dysfunction
- Absence of CN abnormalities

BROWN-SÉQUARD SYNDROME

Brown-Séquard syndrome is commonly caused by an extramedullary lesion (spinal cord hemisection syndrome) and is characterized by the following:

- Ipsilateral (to the lesion) spastic paresis because of involvement of the lateral corticospinal tract
- Ipsilateral lower motor neuron weakness because of involvement of anterior horn cells or roots
- Ipsilateral loss of vibration and joint position sense because of involvement of the posterior column or spinocerebellar tract

- Contralateral loss of pain and temperature sensation because of involvement of the spinothalamic tract

CONUS MEDULLARIS AND CAUDA EQUINA SYNDROMES

Conus medullaris and cauda equina syndromes are usually caused by a compressive lesion (e.g., tumor, cyst) involving the spinal cord at the level of the **conus** (S3–C1) or **epiconus** (L4–S2) or involving spinal roots at the level of the **cauda equina** (lumbosacral roots below L3). Rarely is either syndrome seen without the other because of anatomic proximity. They are clinically difficult to differentiate, but **cauda equina** syndrome has the following characteristics:

- More gradual onset
- Predominantly unilateral (or bilateral but asymmetric) radicular pain
- More asymmetric weakness of lower extremities
- More asymmetric saddle distribution sensory loss
- Absence of knee and ankle jerks
- Sphincter and sexual dysfunction usually are less severe and occur later

Conus medullaris syndrome should be suspected when the patient presents with bilateral lower extremity weakness, diminished or absent ankle reflexes, symmetric saddle sensory loss, and early sphincter (bowel, bladder) or sexual dysfunction.

UPPER MOTOR NEURON AND LOWER MOTOR NEURON FACIAL WEAKNESS

The upper part of the face (forehead) has bilateral innervation from the corticobulbar tract; the lower face has unilateral innervation from the contralateral corticobulbar tract. Lesions involving the facial nerve or nucleus cause ipsilateral upper (forehead) and lower facial muscle weakness (peripheral CN VII palsy). Lesions involving the corticobulbar tract, above the facial nucleus, cause weakness of the contralateral lower face muscles (CN VII palsy).

TONGUE DEVIATION

Lesions involving the nucleus of the axons of CN XII cause the tongue to deviate toward the site of the lesion.

CEREBELLAR LESIONS

Cerebellar lesions are commonly associated with dystaxia or clumsiness of the hands and legs (limb dystaxia) and brain stem symptoms and signs.

LESIONS AFFECTING ANTERIOR HORN CELLS

Lesions affecting anterior horn cells usually are associated with the following characteristics:

- Asymmetric muscle weakness, distal greater than proximal

- Hypotonia
- Muscle atrophy and fasciculation (later stages)
- Hyporeflexia
- Absence of sensory symptoms or deficit

PERIPHERAL POLYNEUROPATHIES

Peripheral polyneuropathies present with the following characteristics:

- Predominantly distal limb paresthesia, hyperesthesia, dysesthesia, and sensory deficit
- Predominantly distal muscle weakness and atrophy
- Hyporeflexia or areflexia
- Sensory deficit in distribution of involved nerves

RADICULOPATHIES

Radiculopathies usually present with the following:

- Unilateral radicular pain or paresthesia
- Neck or back pain
- Muscle weakness
- Possible atrophy in the distribution of the involved root, and hyporeflexia or areflexia

PLEXOPATHIES

Plexopathies are associated with the following:

- Unilateral motor and sensory deficits in the distribution of more than one root and nerve
- Muscle atrophy (later stages)
- Hyporeflexia or areflexia

HAND-MUSCLE WEAKNESS, ATROPHY

Hand-muscle weakness and atrophy can be caused by any of the following:

- C8–T1 radiculopathy
- Lower trunk brachial plexopathy
- Median and ulnar mononeuropathies (carpal and cubital tunnel syndromes)

In C8–T1 radiculopathy and lower trunk brachial plexopathy, look for Horner's syndrome and sensory deficit in the medial aspect of the forearm. In median and ulnar mononeuropathies, the flexor pollicis longus muscle strength is intact (innervated by the anterior interosseus nerve).

WRISTDROP

Wristdrop is characterized by the following:

- Strength of the triceps and brachioradialis muscles is intact; **posterior interosseus mononeuropathy** with no sensory loss

- Wrist extensors are weak, but only the triceps are spared; **radial nerve lesions** at or above the spiral groove
- Wrist extensors and triceps are weak; **radial nerve lesion at the axilla**
- Weakness of wrist extensors, triceps, and deltoid suggest posterior cord of the **brachial plexus**

SCAPULAR WINGING

Scapular winging **caused by serratus anterior weakness** is characterized by the following:

- Winging at rest
- A medially deviated scapula
- Winging accentuated by arm flexion

Winging **caused by trapezius weakness** is characterized by the following:

- Slight winging at rest
- A laterally deviated scapula
- Winging that is accentuated by abduction of the arm, shoulder lower on affected side

FOOTDROP

Peroneal neuropathy versus L5 radiculopathy, weakness of ankle inversion, flexion of toes (flexor digitorum longus), and extension of great toe (extensor hallucis longus) all suggest L5 radiculopathy, which is often associated with back pain, sensory loss, and absence of ankle jerk.

QUADRICEPS WEAKNESS AND ATROPHY

Femoral neuropathy versus L2–L4 radiculopathy. Thigh adductors are strong in pure femoral neuropathy and weak in L2–L4 radiculopathy.

POSTSYNAPTIC NEUROMUSCULAR JUNCTION DISORDER

Postsynaptic neuromuscular junction disorder is characterized by fluctuating, asymmetric, oculobulbar, and proximal limb weakness and normal muscle tone, bulk, sensation, and reflexes.

PRIMARY MUSCLE DISEASE (MYOPATHY)

Myopathy presents with the following:

- Proximal, often symmetric muscle weakness
- Normal or atrophied muscle
- Normal sensory examination and reflexes

7

Neurodiagnostic Tests and Procedures

This chapter outlines some general guidelines for ordering diagnostic tests and procedures that are used to supplement and extend findings from a neurologic history and physical examination. These tests and procedures are ordered to support clinical impressions or exclude other possibilities.

Each patient should be analyzed individually, and diagnostic tests and procedures should be ordered as the patient's condition requires and not because a particular test or procedure is always called for in the particular condition (i.e., not all patients with dementia need an electroencephalogram [EEG] or lumbar puncture [LP]).

I prefer to order tests that provide the most information and are the **least invasive**. Consider ordering **invasive tests** when they provide high sensitivity and specificity and offer beneficial results for treatment planning. The clinician ordering the tests and procedures should be familiar with them, know how they are done, and be familiar with their risks, limitations, contraindications, indications, sensitivity, and specificity. Then the clinician should explain the process, potential risks, invasiveness, and cost of tests to the patient if it is expensive.

Sometimes it is necessary and justified to repeat a test, because it increases the diagnostic yield (e.g., an EEG in evaluating a seizure disorder).

Provide adequate, pertinent history and physical findings to the consultant performing the diagnostic tests or procedures. Be specific about the purpose of the test. In addition, the clinician ordering the test should review the results with the consultant who performs the test (e.g., review and discuss neuroimaging results with the radiologist). Test results and subsequent plans should then be discussed with the patient and family.

If test results do not correlate with the patient's history and physical examination, further history, and perhaps examination, is needed (retrodiagnosis). Test results do not always correlate with the severity of disease (e.g., magnetic resonance imaging [MRI] findings that do not correlate with severity of multiple sclerosis). Incidental, abnormal test results should be handled individually (e.g., asymptomatic carotid stenosis).

Although diagnostic procedures influence a treatment plan, they should not govern treatment (with few exceptions). Treat the patient's problem, not the laboratory results. For example, when treating a patient with polymyositis or myasthenia gravis, the goal of therapy is to improve the patient's strength, not to address a falling serum creatine kinase level or acetylcholine receptor antibody titer. Tests should be used as an objective guide.

Neurologic diagnostic procedures are useful not only when they show abnormal results, but also when they show normal results. For example, a negative computed tomography (CT) head scan or MRI in a stroke patient suggests subcortical lacunar infarction, and a normal EEG in a demented patient suggests pseudodementia.

Most neurodiagnostic procedures are performed on an outpatient basis (e.g., LP, needle electromyography [EMG], myelography, pharmacologic testing). Only a cerebral angiogram requires short-term hospital admission. Test results' reliability depends not only on the interpreter's qualifications, knowledge, and experience, but also on techniques (personnel, equipment, patient's cooperation).

NEUROIMAGING TECHNIQUES

X-Rays

Order plain spinal x-rays in an initial evaluation of patients with spinal injury or neck and back pain or when spine metastasis is suspected. Skull films rarely are taken.

Computed Tomography

- CT scan, now available in almost all health care centers, identifies abnormal density (hypodense [dark] or hyperdense [white, bright]).

- CT is a good screening neuroimaging technique for the initial assessment of patients with stroke, intracerebral and subarachnoid hemorrhage, head trauma, meningitis, dementia, hydrocephalus, and brain tumors.
- It is superior to MRI for detecting intracerebral hemorrhage, particularly subarachnoid hemorrhage, and calcified lesions. Usually a noncontrast CT scan is sufficient.
- Iodinated contrast agents may be necessary when an enhancing lesion (tumors, vascular malformation, metastasis, inflammatory disease) is suspected.
- CT is less sensitive and specific than MRI; therefore, an MRI, if available, should be ordered in the diagnosis of suspected small central nervous system lesions (e.g. small stroke, lacunae), multiple sclerosis, brain metastasis, primary brain tumors, inflammatory diseases (e.g., vasculitis, herpes encephalitis, acquired immunodeficiency syndrome encephalopathy), brain stem and posterior fossa lesions, pituitary tumors, temporal lobe lesions (e.g., patients with intractable complex partial seizures), spinal cord lesions, and compression.

Magnetic Resonance Imaging

- MRI is more sensitive and specific than CT for detecting brain and spinal cord lesions, and its higher resolution shows detailed anatomy.

- MRI is an ideal neuroimaging technique for assessing sinus venous thrombosis and lesions involving the brain stem, posterior fossa, and spinal cord.
- In T1-weighted MRI, the cerebrospinal fluid appears dark; in T2-weighted MRI the cerebrospinal fluid and eyeballs have a bright white appearance. The T1-weighted image shows outline anatomy; the T2-weighted image is good for imaging pathology. The contrast agent in MRI (gadolinium) is relatively safe and nonionic.
- Contrast MRI is useful in enhancing lesion or detecting disruption of the blood-brain barrier.
- MRI rapidly is replacing many neurodiagnostic tests such as evoked potentials (EPs), myelography, cisternography, CT, and brain scanning.

Following are **some disadvantages of MRI**:

- Expense.
- Nonavailability and limited availability.
- Patients must be cooperative and able to lie still for testing (45 minutes on average).
- Patients requiring close monitoring (e.g., comatose patients) are unsuited for MRI.
- Nonaccommodating for obese patients (weighing more than 300 lbs).
- Claustrophobia in some patients requires presedation.

- Contraindicated in patients with pacemakers, metallic clip (cerebral aneurysm), cochlear implants, Harrington rods, or other metallic foreign bodies.

Myelography

Since the advancement of CT scan and MRI, myelography is rarely used. The procedure involves injecting water-soluble contrast agent into the subarachnoid space. Myelography is an invasive procedure and includes risk of back pain, post-LP headache, infection, and occasionally seizures. Most often, myelography is performed in neurosurgery or orthopedic departments. If an MRI is not available and the condition indicates spinal root and cord compression, myelography followed by CT is reasonable.

Cerebral Angiography

Cerebral angiography, an invasive procedure, is used to view extracranial and intracranial blood vessels. Contrast agent is injected through a catheter into the femoral or brachial artery. Arteriograms are estimated to cause approximately 1% morbidity and mortality. Cerebral angiography is reserved for highly selected cases when CT or MRI provides no definite answers, when vascular lesion (e.g., vasculitis, arteriovenous malformation) or arterial dissection is suspected, or when carotid endarterectomy is contemplated. Arteriography also is used to treat or obliterate arteriovenous malformation by injecting particles (interventional angiography).

Magnetic Resonance Angiography

Magnetic resonance angiography (MRA), a noninvasive technique, is used to view extracranial or intracranial blood vessels and to identify stenosis or blood vessel occlusion. The technique is particularly useful in detecting sinus venous thromboses, arterial dissections, and aneurysms greater than 3 mm in diameter. MRA is a quick, noninvasive screening test for arterial stenosis; however, it is not as sensitive as conventional angiography. It is an alternative to angiography in elderly individuals, patients with renal failure, and patients with an allergy to contrast agent.

Carotid Doppler Ultrasonography

Carotid Doppler ultrasonography, which measures the degree of carotid stenosis according to velocity of blood flow through the blood vessel, is an extremely sensitive, noninvasive procedure used to evaluate carotid stenosis in patients with stroke or transient ischemic attacks (TIAs). It can differentiate between an occluded and an open artery, but the degree of stenosis usually is underestimated with this technique. This technique can be used to determine the need for further studies (e.g., MRA or angiography).

Transcranial Doppler Ultrasonography

Transcranial Doppler (TCD) ultrasonography measures blood flow and noninvasively images the velocity of cerebral circulation in the distribution of major intracranial arteries. In experienced hands, this procedure is safe, fast, and reliable. Use of TCD ultrasonography is **indicated** in the following situations:

- To detect whether stenosis is greater than 50% in major intracranial arteries
- To assess the collateral circulation of intracranial arteries
- To assess and monitor response to treatment of cerebral vasospasm after subarachnoid hemorrhage
- To detect arteriovenous malformations (AVMs) to assess arteries and blood flow involved in the AVM, and to evaluate treatment after embolization (particles injected into the AVM)

TCD may become the procedure of choice to assess brain death and to monitor increased intracranial pressure.

Positron Emission Tomography

Positron emission tomography (PET) is a technique that maps different anatomic regions of the brain according to biochemical, physiologic, or pharmacologic characteristics. CT and MRI image the brain according to structural abnormalities (structural imaging); PET images the brain according to functional abnormalities (functional imaging). PET uses radioisotopes (e.g., oxygen, carbon) produced in a cyclotron, then incorporated into a biological agent. Specific receptor ligands are labeled to map specific receptor sites (e.g., cholinergic, adrenergic, serotonergic). The most commonly used agent for humans is 18F-fluoro-2-deoxy-D-glucose (FDG). Although frequently used as a research tool, PET's clinical use is increasing. FDG-PET is a safe, sensitive technique with limited use because of cost, technical complexity (requiring a cyclotron), and unavailability. Following are current clinical uses of PET:

- To localize epileptogenic focus in patients considered for surgical treatment of epilepsy (intractable) seizure
- To differentiate diagnosis of Alzheimer's disease from multi-infarct dementia
- To confirm early diagnosis of Parkinson's disease or Huntington's disease or to differentiate Parkinson's disease from progressive supranuclear palsy
- To grade primary brain tumor and choose the site for biopsy
- To differentiate postirradiation brain necrosis (encephalopathy) from recurrent brain tumor (PET is probably the best test to differentiate these two conditions.)

Single-Photon Emission Computed Tomography

Single-photon emission CT (SPECT) measures regional cerebral blood flow, which correlates with regional cerebral metabolism. A radioisotope is tagged with a receptor-binding agent and injected intravenously. The common agent is Tc-hexamethylpropylene amine oxime, which crosses the blood-brain barrier and metabolizes to a less lipophilic compound and leaves the brain slowly; therefore, regional cerebral blood flow can be measured for several hours. SPECT does not require a cyclotron, and the radioisotope is available commercially. The cost of a SPECT scan is comparable to that of a CT scan, and SPECT is more widely available than PET. The indications for SPECT are the same as for PET.

ELECTROPHYSIOLOGIC TESTS

Nerve Conduction Studies and Needle Electromyography

Although the term *EMG* is used in practice, it actually is two procedures—a **nerve conduction study (NCS)** and **needle EMG**. EMG is used to evaluate **motor unit** integrity and dysfunction (the motor unit being a single motor nerve and all muscle fibers it innervates). In broader terms, the motor unit consists of the anterior horn cell, root, plexus, peripheral nerves, neuromuscular junction, and muscle fibers (peripheral nervous system [PNS]). EMG is the single most useful diagnostic test to assess diseases of the PNS.

Nerve Conduction Studies

NCSs are performed by either a physician or a qualified, trained technician. Any accessible nerve can be stimulated. NCS consists of **motor nerve conduction (MNC) studies** and **sensory nerve conduction (SNC) studies.**

For MNC studies, the nerve is stimulated by a surface electrode at different sites along the nerve (usually two sites), and the motor nerve action potential or compound motor action potential (CMAP) is recorded from a surface electrode placed over the motor point of the innervated muscle. Needle electrodes rarely are used for stimulation or recording. **Latency** (time required for the nerve impulse from stimulation site to produce an action potential), **amplitude** (height of action potential), **morphology**, and **conduction velocity** (the velocity between the stimulating sites) are measured. Detectable abnormalities for motor and sensory nerves include conduction block, absence of response, slowing of conduction velocity, delayed latencies, decreasing amplitude, and change in morphology.

For **SNC** studies, the mixed or purely sensory nerves (i.e., sural, superficial radial) are stimulated and sensory nerve action potential (SNAP) is recorded from the skin nerve. Measuring SNAPs are particularly useful in evaluating patients with suspected peripheral polyneuropathies, focal neuropathies (e.g., carpal tunnel syndrome), plexopathy, and sensory neuronopathy (diseases affecting dorsal root ganglia).

Needle Electromyography

Needle EMG is performed only by a physician (neurologist or physiatrist). A disposable needle (concentric) inserted into the muscle measures impulses during rest and at minimum and maximum voluntary contraction. During rest a normal muscle is "quiet" and does not produce any sound or waves (except when the needle is inserted at the end-plate region). Abnormal activities at rest include the following reactions:

- **Fibrillation potentials** (related to a single muscle fiber)
- **Fasciculations** (potentials from several muscle fibers)
- **Positive sharp waves** (a downward deflected wave form) and repetitive complex discharges

Motor unit potentials, produced by a group of muscle fibers belonging to a corresponding motor neuron, are used to differentiate **neuropathic** from **myopathic** (muscle disease) disorders and are evaluated during voluntary minimal contraction. The **morphology**, **amplitude**, **duration**, **number** of phases, and **complexity** of the wave form are then assessed.

Indications

NCS and needle EMG should be ordered when any of the following are suspected: motor neuron disease (e.g., amyotrophic lateral sclerosis), radiculopathy (neck and back pain), plexopathy, peripheral polyneuropathy, entrapment neuropathy (e.g., carpal tunnel syndrome), nerve injury (e.g., from gunshot wounds), neuromuscular junction disorders (e.g., myasthenia gravis, myasthenic syndrome, botulism), and primary muscle disease (e.g., inflammatory myopathies, muscular dystrophy, metabolic myopathy).

The electromyographer should acquire a pertinent history and physical findings to obtain the best results from an EMG.

Complications and Limitations

Although needle EMG is invasive, it is a safe, sensitive, specific test and causes only minor discomfort for most patients. Most patients tolerate this procedure. Because the needles used are disposable, the risk of infectious disease transmission is virtually nonexistent. The EMG sensitivity depends on the duration, stage, and severity of the suspected disease; extent of the study performed; and the electromyographer's knowledge and experience.

Other Techniques

Repetitive Nerve Stimulation

Repetitive nerve stimulation is a technique used to detect neuromuscular junction disorders (e.g., **myasthenia gravis**, **Lambert-Eaton syndrome**). CMAPs are recorded from a distal or proximal muscle; then the nerve is stimulated at the rate of two times per second. A gradual decrease of CMAP amplitude is decrement, which is considered abnormal if it exceeds 10%. In presynaptic disorders (e.g., myasthenic syndrome), there is significant amplitude increase (increment) when the nerve is stimulated at a higher rate (greater than 20 times per second) or after brief muscle exercise followed by a single shock stimulation.

Single-Fiber Electromyography
Single-fiber EMG is a highly specialized, time-consuming technique performed only by an experienced electromyographer. This procedure is indicated when myasthenia gravis is suspected and repetitive nerve stimulation and antibody measurement are inconclusive. In this technique, a pair of muscle fibers that belong to one anterior horn cell is isolated with minimal voluntary muscle contraction. The pair of muscle fibers usually fire at the same time, but in myasthenia gravis and myasthenic syndrome they fire irregularly (known as *jitter*). Single-fiber EMG is highly sensitive but nonspecific. In neuromuscular diseases and neurogenic and myopathic conditions, jitter is increased compared with normal.

Evoked Potentials

EPs are used to assess the integrity of sensory pathways in the central nervous system. The mixed or sensory nerve is stimulated repeatedly and responses are recorded through surface electrodes placed on the spine or cerebral cortex. The responses are computer averaged (deleting background noise and extracting EEG). Measuring EPs is noninvasive but ordered less frequently because of the use of MRI. Abnormalities revealed by EPs indicate a lesion on the same side of the brain (side-to-side abnormalities are assessed). EP yields less specific results regarding etiology; therefore, findings should be interpreted within the context of clinical features.

Visual Evoked Potentials

With visual EPs, the unilateral retina is stimulated by having the patient look at a changing black-and-white checkerboard pattern (pattern reversal stimuli). Recording electrodes are placed over the occipital head regions. The major positive wave (P100) occurs after approximately 100 milliseconds. A unilateral abnormality of P100 (prolonged latency) indicates optic nerve lesion anterior to the optic chiasm (e.g., optic neuritis). Bilateral abnormalities of P100 (delayed latency, decreased amplitude, or absence of response) suggests a lesion affecting the visual pathways from the retina, optic nerves anterior to the chiasm, or optic tracts behind the chiasm.

Indications

- Patients suspected of having multiple sclerosis
- Functional vision loss

Brain Stem Auditory Evoked Potentials

With brain stem auditory EPs, the unilateral (monaural) auditory nerve is stimulated by a constant clicking sound while the other ear is masked by white noise. Commonly, five waves (waves I, II, III, IV, V) are measured in the first 10 milliseconds. The more reliable, stable waves are waves I, III, and V. The parameters measured include the absolute latencies of each wave and interpeak latencies of waves I–III, III–V, and I–V, as well as amplitude. A prolonged interpeak latency of III–V suggests a pontomesencephalic lesion.

Indications

- Diagnosing multiple sclerosis
- Diagnosing posterior fossa tumor, acoustic neuroma, and cerebellopontine angle lesions
- Confirming brain death
- Evaluating hearing in normal children or in children after meningitis

Somatosensory Evoked Potentials

Somatosensory EPs are an extension of NCS. The peripheral nerve (median, ulnar, peroneal, or tibialis) is stimulated repeatedly. Responses, recorded from the spine (dorsal column) and somatosensory cortex (vertex head region), are varied depending on the height of the patient and limb length.

Indications

- Diagnosing multiple sclerosis
- Diagnosing subacute combined degeneration

- Diagnosing spinocerebellar degeneration and spinal cord trauma
- Diagnosing functional hemisensory loss
- Monitoring spinal cord function during spine surgery (prime use in recent years)

Electroencephalography

EEG records spontaneous brain potentials from approximately 21 pairs of electrodes placed over the scalp. The electrodes are interconnected montages. The EEG is assessed during wakeful and resting stages, as well as during active **hyperventilation**, **sleep**, and **photic stimulation** procedures. The EEG is recorded as an analog on EEG paper or as digital on a disk. In special circumstances, an EEG can be recorded continuously using an ambulatory cassette and prolonged video EEG monitoring.

Clinicians should know the normal EEG wave forms, which are distinguished from each other by their morphology, frequency (measured by hertz), location, and reactivity. Following are brief descriptions of the wave forms:

- Alpha (8–13 Hz)—located over parieto-occipital head regions, present during wakefulness, enhanced by eye closing, and disappear with eye opening
- Beta (more than 13 Hz)
- Theta (4–7 Hz)—occur normally during sleep; their presence is abnormal during wakefulness

- Delta (1–3 Hz)—occur normally during deeper sleep and their presence is abnormal during wakefulness

Many abnormalities recorded by EEG are nonspecific, with few exceptions (vide infra). The main abnormal waves in EEG are slow waves (theta and delta while awake) and epileptiform discharges (spike and sharp waves).

Electroencephalography in Epilepsy

EEG is used to differentiate epilepsy from nonepileptic events (e.g., syncope, TIA), to differentiate partial from generalized epilepsy (classification), and to help diagnose specific epileptic syndromes.

A Few Specific Epileptic Patterns

- Hypsarrhythmia: infantile spasm
- 3-Hz spike and wave discharge: absence
- Generalized slow-spike and wave: Lennox-Gastaut syndrome
- Generalized multiple spike and wave: myoclonic epilepsy
- Periodic lateralized epileptiform discharges (PLEDs): herpes simplex, encephalitis, acute infarct, metastasis

Caveat: The most conclusive evidence of epilepsy is gained by recording a clinical seizure simultaneously with epileptic discharges in an EEG (i.e., electroclinical seizure or ictal event); however, most outpatient EEGs are recorded **interictally** (between the seizures). Therefore, a normal EEG does not exclude epilepsy.

Electroencephalography in Status Epilepticus

Continuous EEG recording is done in many centers for patients with status epilepticus. EEG is also particularly useful for

- **Nonconvulsive status epilepticus** (absence or complex partial)
- Suspected ongoing **electrical status** (seizure) in patients with grand mal status when clinical motor convulsions have stopped

Electroencephalography in Alteration of Mental State

Alteration of mental state usually produces generalized, slow waves. Some metabolic encephalopathies may be associated with sharp, triphasic waves (hepatic).

Hint: If a patient is confused and disoriented but the EEG shows only minimal slowing, suspect degenerative disorder. If a patient is less confused, but the EEG shows significant slowing and sharp waves, suspect metabolic encephalopathy (EEG is worse than patient).

Electroencephalography in Coma

An EEG is particularly useful for making a prognosis in a comatose patient. For example, alpha-coma, burst-suppression pattern, iso-electric, and periodic pattern indicate poor prognosis.

Electroencephalography in Infection

Irregular EEG wave form patterns can indicate infections, such as the following:

- Herpes simplex encephalitis, indicated by PLEDs (serial recordings may be needed)
- Subacute sclerosing panencephalitis, indicted by periodic (5–8 seconds) bursts of 2–3 Hz high voltage with slow, sharp waves followed by a relatively flat background between
- Creutzfeldt-Jakob disease, indicated by periodic, generalized 1- to 2-Hz sharp, triphasic waves over low amplitude and slow background

Electroencephalography in Pseudoepilepsy

In patients with suspected psychogenic seizures (pseudoepilepsy), the more reliable method of testing is prolonged video and EEG monitoring. Also, an EEG can be monitored during a clinical seizure, which can be induced or suggested.

Electroencephalography in Epilepsy Surgery

For a patient with intractable seizures, prolonged video and EEG monitoring is particularly useful when surgical intervention (e.g., temporal lobectomy) is considered.

Electroencephalography in Brain Death

EEG is used to confirm brain death. EEG is iso-electric when no activity of greater than 2 µv is recorded for 30 minutes. The recording should be performed according to an established protocol. Severe hypothermia, severe hypotension, and intoxication with sedative-hypnotics should be excluded.

Sleep Studies

Polysomnogram

Polysomnogram (PSG) consists of the continuous recording of multiple biological variables (EEG, eye movements, electrocardiography [ECG], submental and limb EMG, respiration, and finger oximetry) during nocturnal sleep. These variables are measured during the awake stage, stages I–IV of non-REM sleep and REM sleep.

Indications

- Insomnia
- Sleep apnea
- Narcolepsy
- Periodic limb movements during sleep
- Idiopathic hypersomnia
- REM behavior sleep disorder
- Parasomnias: sleepwalking, night terrors, nightmares

Multiple Sleep Latency Test

The optimum time for a multiple sleep latency test (MSLT) is after an overnight PSG. Five 20-minute naps are measured every 2 hours for onset of stage I sleep. Sleep-onset REM also is measured. EEG, submental EMG, eye movements, ECG, and respiration are monitored. The average latency of five naps is 10 minutes or longer. Latency of 3–5 minutes is abnormal; latency of 7–8 minutes is borderline. If one nap latency is equal to or greater than 10 minutes, the test is terminated, and five naps are not recorded.

MSLT is indicated in the diagnosis of excessive daytime hypersomnolence and narcolepsy, which calls for a short MSLT or two or more sleep-onset REM measurements.

Autonomic Function Tests

Autonomic function tests (AFTs) assess the integrity of unmyelinated or small myelinated peripheral nerve fibers, which are unmeasurable with conventional NCSs.

Autonomic dysfunction generally presents with symptoms or signs related to **eyes** or **cardiovascular**, **gastrointestinal**, or **genitourinary systems**. AFTs should not be ordered routinely and should be considered only when strongly indicated after a detailed history and physical examination.

In clinical use, tests should be noninvasive, simple, safe, reliable, and reproducible. Most autonomic laboratories (primarily academic) use a battery of familiar tests to evaluate end-organ response to different maneuvers (reflex), which include cardiovagal heart rate response, adrenergic, and sudomotor tests. These tests are safe and noninvasive, with only occasional reports of syncope (during tilt) and minor local skin injuries (during the thermoregulatory sweat test [TsT]). Asking the patient to perform a Valsalva's maneuver may carry some risks in elderly patients (glaucoma) and should not be performed in patients with chronic lung disease. Autonomic tests should be done as a battery; a single test is inadequate. Patients should not be dehydrated or on medications that may affect test results. Following are the battery's test categories:

- **Cardiovagal heart rate response:** Beat-to-beat heart rate variability is measured continuously (by Finapres or Collins monitor) in response to deep breathing, standing, and Valsalva's maneuver.
- **Adrenergic tests:** Beat-to-beat BP is measured during standing, tilt, Valsalva's maneuver, sustained hand grip, or ice cold immersion test.
- **Sudomotor tests:** These tests include quantitative sudomotor axon reflex test, sympathetic skin response, TsT, and sweat imprint.

These tests are indicated in the following conditions:

- Progressive autonomic neuropathy, diabetic neuropathy, amyloid neuropathy, immune-mediated neuropathy, pure autonomic neuropathy, porphyria, Fabry's disease, multiple system atrophy
- Distal small fiber neuropathy
- Postural tachycardia syndrome
- Sympathetically mediated pain
- Syncope
- Evaluation of the response to therapy, such as in patients with diabetes, syncope, Lambert-Eaton myasthenic syndrome (response to 3,4-diaminopyridine)
- Disorders affecting sweat production

LUMBAR PUNCTURE

LP is the insertion of a special needle into the subarachnoid space at L3–L4 or L4–L5 vertebrae for **diagnostic**, **therapeutic**, and **anesthetic** purposes. Because LP is an invasive procedure, the patient's condition must strongly indicate its use.

Before ordering the procedure, the clinician must thoroughly explain to the patient the procedure, risks, purpose, and possible results. Patients typically are nervous, and many have heard about big needles and paralysis. Assure the patient that the procedure is safe—that the thin needle does not touch the spinal cord nor cause paralysis. A patient with suspected bleeding disorders should be evaluated with coagulation studies (prothrombin, partial thromboplastin time, platelet count) before LP is considered. In cases of suspected brain mass or increased intracranial pressure, it is recommended to obtain a head CT scan or MRI before LP.

Indications

Diagnostic Indications

- Central nervous system infections (e.g., meningitis, encephalitis)
- Subarachnoid hemorrhage
- Demyelinating disorders (e.g., multiple sclerosis)
- Inflammatory polyneuropathies (e.g., Guillain-Barré syndrome, chronic inflammatory demyelinating polyneuropathy)
- Paraneoplastic syndrome
- Unexplained dementia with progressive course and acute onset
- Vasculitis (e.g., stroke in young)
- Pseudotumor cerebri (to measure opening pressure)
- Normal pressure hydrocephalus (to predict the response to shunt)
- Myelography (with or without CT scan)

Therapeutic Indications

- **Intrathecal administration of medications** (e.g., antibiotic or antifungal agent, chemotherapy agent, antispastic agent, pain medication)
- Relieving pressure (e.g., pseudotumor)
- Blood patch for treatment of post-LP headaches.

Anesthetic Indications

LP is also an anesthetic tool for epidural block for pain management or during delivery.

Procedure

The procedure for administering an LP is as follows:

1. Request a nurse to assist in the procedure.
2. Expose the patient's lower back and hip.
3. Mark anatomic landmark.
4. Clean the area widely.
5. Position the patient in the fetal position on his or her left lateral decubitus.
6. Position yourself comfortably.
7. Insert the needle between the L3 and L4 interspace; the needle plane should be vertical, with the bevel facing up.
8. Direct the needle toward the umbilicus.
9. When you feel a pop, draw the stylet, and let one drop of fluid escape, then always measure the

pressure by extending the patient's legs out of the fetal position.

10. If you fail to obtain cerebrospinal fluid ("dry tap"), consider the following options: Insert the needle slightly deeper, rotate the needle, aspirate very slowly, consider putting the patient in a sitting position, ask a colleague to try, or perform the LP under fluoroscopy.

11. Obtain an adequate amount of fluid. In addition, save, label, and freeze one tube (2 ml) for future reference.

In a suspected traumatic bloody tap, take the following precautions:

- Gradual clearing should be noted from first tube to last.
- A bloody tap caused by trauma does not clot.
- Fluid should be processed in a centrifuge.
- The ratio of white blood cells to red blood cells in a traumatic tap is approximately 1:700.
- A traumatic tap is not associated with high cerebrospinal fluid protein concentration.

Contraindications

- Increased intracranial pressure except in pseudotumor cerebri
- When platelet count is less than 20,000, or when the patient is on anticoagulant therapy

- Subcutaneous infection at the site of insertion
- Complete spinal cord block caused by mass (e.g., Froin's syndrome), which shows extremely high cerebrospinal fluid protein concentration

Complications

- Iatrogenic post-LP meningitis
- Post-LP headaches (e.g., headache on standing, common in women, occurs in approximately 10–15% of cases beginning 3–5 days after LP and resolving spontaneously. In chronic post-LP headache, a blood patch gives immediate, dramatic relief.)
- Bleeding (e.g., spinal epidural, subdural, subarachnoid)
- Transient unilateral sixth nerve palsy
- Backache
- Occasional transient lower limb paresthesia
- Brain herniation in cases of supra- or subtentorial mass

BIOPSIES

Brain Biopsy

Brain biopsy is considered when all noninvasive methods fail to provide a diagnosis. Brain biopsy is considered particularly in younger patients when the diagnosis may influence the treatment and also enhance prognosis. Most brain biopsies are done by stereotaxis technique. Complications include hemorrhage, infection, and neurologic deficit.

Brain biopsy is indicated in the diagnosis of primary brain tumor or single metastasis, infection such as herpes simplex encephalitis, and degenerative disorders of the brain such as suspected cases of Creutzfeldt-Jakob disease.

Ideally, **brain biopsy is performed when the lesion site** can be localized by imaging techniques, when the lesion is superficial and accessible, and when no critical brain region (language zone) or the brain stem is involved.

Leptomeningeal Biopsy

Leptomeningeal biopsy is performed in cases of highly suspected isolated central nervous system vasculitis or carcinomatous meningitis.

Temporal Artery Biopsy

Temporal artery biopsy is used in the diagnosis of suspected cases of temporal arteritis.

Muscle Biopsy

Muscle biopsy is performed—using an incision or needle—on an outpatient basis, with the patient under local anesthesia. Muscle biopsy has minimal risk of infection, bruising, and discomfort. The muscle to be biopsied should be selected from weak, but not wasted, muscles. Muscle biopsy is indicated for any myogenic (myopathy) disease such as polymyositis, metabolic and mitochon-

drial myopathies, muscular dystrophies, or congenital
myopathies.

Nerve Biopsy

Nerve biopsy is commonly performed under local anesthesia from the sural nerve behind the lateral malleolus.
The obtained biopsy specimen must be processed ade-
quately in a reliable, experienced laboratory. A nerve
biopsy is indicated in unexplained peripheral polyneuropathies when all diagnostic tests have been exhausted.

   The main indications for a nerve biopsy are vasculitic
neuropathies, amyloid neuropathy, inflammatory neuropathy, leprosy, and storage neuropathies (e.g., meta-
chromatic leukodystrophy). The side effects of a nerve
biopsy are hypersensitivity and discomfort at the site of
the biopsy, which often resolve spontaneously after several weeks.

ISCHEMIC EXERCISE FOREARM TEST

The ischemic exercise forearm test is considered in
patients presenting with postexertional myalgia, particularly when McArdle's disease (myophosphorylase deficiency) or deaminase deficiency is suspected. Baseline
serum lactate and ammonia concentrations are measured.
Ischemia is induced by using a blood pressure cuff to
raise the blood pressure above systolic level. The patient
then exercises by continuously squeezing a hand grip

ergometer for 1–2 minutes. The blood pressure cuff is released and blood from the antecubital vein is dawn. Serum lactate and ammonia concentrations are measured 0, 3, 5, 10, and 15 minutes after exercise. No rise in lactate or ammonia concentrations when compared with baseline and a control subject is considered abnormal.

PHARMACOLOGIC TESTS

Edrophonium (Tensilon) Test

The Tensilon test is used to diagnosis myasthenia gravis. It is done in an outpatient setting, except for elderly patients and patients with history of chronic lung disease or cardiac history, when it is recommended the test be done as an inpatient or in the emergency room with continuous monitoring.

The total test dose is 10 mg/ml: 2 mg are administered as a test dose; the remaining 8 mg is administered as a unit or in increments. A clear, objective muscle weakness (e.g., ptosis, eye muscle weakness, dysarthria) must be established before a Tensilon test is performed. False-positive results occur when a clear objective deficit cannot be established (e.g., fatigue).

Cocaine Test

The cocaine test is used to localize the lesion site in Horner's syndrome. One drop of 10% cocaine is instilled into each eye, followed by another drop 1 minute later. Both eyes should dilate in approximately 45 minutes. The pupil with loss of sympathetic innervation (Horner's) will not dilate. To further localize the lesion, one drop of 1% hydroxyamphetamine (Paredrine test) is instilled in both eyes. Normal pupils will not dilate; the side affected by Horner's syndrome dilates, which indicates a first- or second-order neuron as the site of the lesion.

Common Neurologic Conditions

Common Neurologic Conditions

8

Stroke

EMERGENCY ROOM TREATMENT OF STROKE

Initial Assessment for Stroke on Arrival

When the patient arrives in the emergency room and is suspected of having a stroke do the following:

- Stabilize the patient's vitals and monitor heart and blood pressure (BP).
- Start an intravenous (IV) line and administer 25% normal saline at a rate of 50–75 ml per hour.
- Send a blood sample to the laboratory for a complete blood cell count, prothrombin time, partial thromboplastin time, platelet count, and chemistry profile.
- Obtain a 12-lead electrocardiogram.
- Obtain a brief, pertinent medical and neurologic history and establish onset and duration of stroke.
- Do a 5-minute neurologic examination focusing on mental status, pupillary function, stiff neck, and focal neurologic deficits.

- Consult the hospital's neurologist and stroke team.
- Obtain a computed tomography (CT) head scan without contrast to exclude hemorrhagic stroke or mass lesion.

Therapeutic Considerations

- Administer oxygen.
- Elevate the patient's head to approximately 30 degrees.
- Consider a thrombolytic agent such as tissue plasminogen activator (tPA), which should be given within 3 hours of ischemic stroke. Consult a neurologist, stroke specialist, or emergency room physician for confirmation. Strictly follow protocol guidelines.
- Treat any seizure with an antiepileptic drug.
- Avoid administering fluid containing glucose. If the patient's blood glucose level is elevated, try to normalize it within 6 hours (high glucose levels are associated with poor outcome).

Elevated Blood Pressure

What You Should Know

- In acute stroke, systemic arterial BP often is elevated. Most patients with stroke are hypertensive. In most cases this elevation is transient and self-limited, and it is caused by autonomic overactivity in an acute setting.

- In acute ischemic stroke, the patient has partial or complete loss of autoregulation; therefore, regional cerebral blood flow depends on systemic arterial BP to maintain adequate perfusion.
- In acute stroke, the peri-infarct penumbra zone is ischemic, but it has functional neural tissue and rapidly lowering BP, causing further ischemia (deteriorating stroke).

What You Should Do

- Generally, no treatment is necessary for mild to moderately elevated BP.
- Antihypertensive drug treatment can be held temporarily in hypertensive patients with mildly elevated BP. Check BP several times before treatment. If treatment is necessary, it should be done slowly and neurologic functions monitored.
- In acute stroke, **hypertension treatment is considered in the following situations**:
  - For patients with hemorrhagic stroke
  - For patients with BP of more than 220/130 mm Hg or mean arterial BP is greater than 130 mm Hg
  - For patients with papilledema
  - For patients with dissecting aneurysm
  - For patients with end-organ dysfunction (e.g., cardiac ischemia or renal failure)
  - When tPA treatment is considered

- In a severely hypertensive patient, the target BP is 185/105–110 mm Hg.
- Ideal antihypertensive drug therapy in an acute setting should be parenteral, easy to titrate, slow acting, and should not raise intracranial pressure.
- The two most commonly used agents are angiotensin-converting enzyme inhibitors (enalapril) and beta blockers (labetalol). A calcium antagonist (nifedipine) is not recommended. Labetalol is given IV at a rate of 10 mg, with an increase of 10 mg every 20 minutes thereafter up to 300 mg, then 10 mg every 8 hours if necessary. This drug cannot be used in patients with diabetes or asthma.

Further Assessment, Workup, and Management

Further Assessment

1. Admit the patient for close observation of vital signs and neurologic functions.
2. Obtain a more detailed history, including onset of stroke, time and occurrence of stroke, duration and evolution of stroke, and preceding symptoms (e.g., headache, transient ischemic attack [TIA], transient vision loss).
3. Establish the medical history of risk factors such as previous stroke or TIA, hypertension, diabetes, heart disease, peripheral vascular disease, high cholesterol, drug abuse, and smoking.

4. Complete the examination with special attention to
   the following:
   - **Neurovascular examination:**
     - Record the patient's BP on both arms and on
       separate occasions.
     - Note the peripheral pulses.
     - Listen for carotid and subclavicular bruits.
     - Listen for a heart murmur or arrhythmia.
     - Examine the patient's fundi for papilledema,
       retinopathy, or retinal emboli.
   - **Neurologic examination:** Complete the neuro-
     logic examination and try to answer the follow-
     ing questions:
     - **What is the location of the stroke** (e.g., corti-
       cal or subcortical)?
     - **What blood supply to the brain is affected**
       (e.g., anterior or posterior circulation, large or
       small blood vessels)?
     - Is the stroke **ischemic** or **hemorrhagic**?
     - Which part of brain is **involved** and which
       part is **spared**?

Workup

Table 8-1 presents the **workup** that most neurologists recommend for patients with stroke or TIA.

Table 8.1 Stroke and Transient Ischemic Attack Workup

Organ	Routine	Selective
Brain	Computed tomogram, magnetic resonance image	Electroencephalogram, single photon emission computed tomogram
Heart	Electrocardiogram, chest x-ray, echocardiogram	Holter monitor, cardiac scan, thallium scan, transesophageal echocardiogram
Blood vessel	Carotid Doppler ultrasound	Magnetic resonance angiogram/cerebral angiogram
Blood	Complete blood cell count, prothrombin time, partial thromboplastin time, lipid profile, erythrocyte sedimentation rate, fluorescent treponemal antibody	Protein culture and sensitivity, antithrombin III, antiphospholipid antibodies, homocysteine, other coagulation factors

Further Management

A. Ischemic brain edema. Cerebral edema after ischemic stroke peaks approximately 48–72 hours after the onset of stroke. Cerebral edema with raised intercranial pressure and transtentorial herniation is a common cause of acute mortality in stroke patients. **Ischemic brain edema** begins as cytotoxic and changes to vasogenic. Treatment and prevention should include the following:
   1. Provide supplemental oxygen.
   2. Elevate the patient's head to 30 degrees.

3. Intubate and hyperventilate the patient briefly to a $Paco_2$ of 25–30 mm Hg if the patient scores less than 8 on the Glasgow Coma Scale.

4. Administer hyperosmolar agents (mannitol [20%] at a rate of 1 g/kg over 30 minutes, followed by 0.25 g per kilogram, every 4–6 hours). Follow with clinical response and serum osmolality.

5. Try furosemide 40 mg IV two times a day.

6. Restrict fluids.

7. Use caution in administering steroids. The effects of using steroids have not been established.

8. Consider surgical intervention such as hemicraniectomy and decompression in a patient with a large cerebellar infarct or a young patient with a large ischemic stroke and deteriorating neurologic status.

B. Complications of stroke. Prevent and treat **complications of stroke**, including aspiration pneumonia, urinary tract infection, deep venous thrombosis, decubiti, hyperglycemia, and cardiac arrhythmia.

C. Risk factors for stroke. Modify **risk factors for stroke**, which include hypertension, diabetes, cardiac disease, cardiac arrhythmia, high cholesterol, and cigarette smoking.

Preventive Measures for Stroke

Medical prevention measures include the following therapies:

- **Antiplatelet** administration—aspirin, 80–1,300 mg per day; ticlopidine, 250 mg twice a day; clopidogrel, 75 mg per day; or combination of aspirin and dipyridamole.
- **Anticoagulant** administration—heparin followed by warfarin. Indications include cardiogenic embolization, stroke in evolution, coagulopathy, carotid dissection.

   Surgical prevention measures include carotid endarterectomy for high-grade stenosis (more than 79% by angiogram).

TRANSIENT ISCHEMIC ATTACKS

- TIAs are sudden neurologic deficits that resolve spontaneously and completely within 24 hours (usually within 15–20 minutes).
- They are a major risk factor for stroke and heart attack: The incidence of ischemic stroke is approximately 10% after TIAs.
- Patients who have experienced recent TIAs (within 7–10 days), crescendo TIAs (series), or prolonged TIAs (duration of several hours) should be admitted to a hospital to expedite workup and management.

- TIAs usually are caused by embolization from artery to artery (e.g., carotid to middle cerebral artery) or from heart to artery (cardiogenic). Other causes include vasculopathies, hematologic diseases, and steal syndrome.
- Patients with lateralized and stereotyped (same distribution) repeated TIAs usually have artery-to-artery embolization.
- If hemispheric TIAs are associated with amaurosis fugax (transient monocular blindness), suspect an internal carotid source for embolization.
- Individuals who are at high risk of TIA include those who have experienced frequent attacks, elderly males, those with active heart disease, and those who have peripheral vascular disease.
- Consider TIA when an elderly individual presents with transient neurologic symptoms and signs.
- TIAs should be differentiated from complicated migraine, partial seizure, syncope, lacunar infarct, multiple sclerosis, and carpal tunnel syndrome.
- The workup for patients with TIAs is the same as for patients with stroke (see Table 8-1). Patients who seek treatment within 72 hours of TIA onset should be hospitalized. Patients seeking treatment after 7 days or more of onset can reasonably be treated on an outpatient basis.

- Treatment of TIAs includes modification of risk factors and preventive measures (e.g., use of antiplatelets [aspirin, ticlopidine, clopidogrel] or anticoagulants [warfarin]). Surgical preventive treatment includes carotid endarterectomy.

LACUNAR STROKE

Lacunar infarcts are small, ischemic strokes in the distribution of small penetrating arteries of the circle of Willis (lenticulostriate, thalamoperforate) and paramedian branches of the basilar artery. The common locations of lacunae are the internal capsule, basal ganglia, thalamus, and pons. Lacunar infarcts account for approximately 20% of all ischemic strokes.

When Lunar Stroke Should be Suspected

Suspect lunar stroke when
- The arms and legs are equally affected (motor or sensory deficit).
- Motor or sensory deficit occurs that is not associated with higher cortical function abnormalities such as aphasia, apraxia, astereognosis, and agraphesthesia.
- Dense neurologic deficit occurs associated with normal repeated CT scan of the head.

Risk Factors for Lacunar Stroke

- Hypertension

- Diabetes
- Hypercholesterolemia
- Aging
- Smoking

Common Clinical Lacunar Syndromes

- Pure motor hemiplegia (posterior limb of internal capsule or pons infarct)
- Pure sensory (thalamic infarct)
- Dysarthria, or clumsy hand (internal capsule or pons infarct)
- Leg paresis and ataxia (pons or internal capsule infarct)

Workup, Prognosis, and Treatment for Lacunar Stroke

Workup for lacunar stroke is same as for stroke (see Table 8-1). Cerebral angiogram generally is not indicated unless carotid endarterectomy is considered. Prognosis of lacunar stroke is generally good. Treatment is the same as for other ischemic strokes, with the exception of anticoagulation (heparin, warfarin), which is rarely indicated.

EMBOLIC STROKE

Embolic (as opposed to thrombotic) stroke should be suspected when the following conditions are observed:

- The patient has sudden, fixed neurologic deficit, particularly during the daytime and activity.

- The patient's neurologic deficit resolves rapidly (sudden onset and offset).
- The stroke is associated with headache, seizure, or altered mental status.
- The stroke occurs in young adults.
- The stroke occurs in the distribution of two or more major blood vessels of the brain (not in the distribution of a penetrating blood vessel).
- The stroke occurs in a patient with a strong **history of heart disease** but weak history of atherosclerosis (documented by history and diagnostic tests).
- Hemorrhagic infarct is demonstrated on CT head scan.
- The patient has acute isolated neurologic deficits such as aphasia or visual field defect.

A **strong history of heart disease** includes atrial fibrillation, valvular disease, myocardial infarction, cardiomyopathy, prosthetic valves, ventricular hypokinesia or dilatation, cardiac thrombus, atrial myxoma, and patent foramen ovale (paradoxical embolization).

SPONTANEOUS INTRACEREBRAL HEMORRHAGE

Spontaneous intracerebral hemorrhage is caused by the following conditions:

- Ruptured cerebral aneurysm or arteriovenous malformation.

- Hypertensive hemorrhage commonly occurs in the pons, basal ganglia, and thalamus.
- Drugs (cocaine, amphetamines).
- Anticoagulant administration (warfarin).
- Thrombocytopenia or other coagulopathies.
- Cerebral amyloid angiopathy in elderly patients; presents with recurrent lobar hemorrhage.
- Central nervous system (CNS) vasculitis.
- Metastasis (melanoma, renal cell carcinoma, lung cancer, choriocarcinoma).

Caveat: Knowing the location of the hemorrhage helps establish the cause. CT scan of the head is superior to magnetic resonance imaging (MRI) in detecting intracerebral hemorrhage. It is imperative to establish the cause of hemorrhage. Consult a neurosurgeon; many hematomas can be evacuated. Surgical evacuation of a cerebellar hemorrhage can be life saving. Consider treating elevated BP more aggressively in hemorrhagic stroke. Stabilize the patient's airway and treat increased intracranial pressure.

SUBARACHNOID HEMORRHAGE

- The two leading causes of spontaneous subarachnoid hemorrhage (SAH) are ruptured saccular aneurysm and arteriovenous malformation.
- Most cerebral aneurysms (saccular, berry) occur in the anterior circulation distribution (30% in anterior com-

municating artery, 24% in posterior communicating artery, and 13% in middle cerebral artery).

- The incidence of SAH aneurysm is approximately 10 per 100,000 per year.
- CT scan of the head is the preferred neuroimaging procedure to document hemorrhage. If the CT head scan is negative, perform a lumbar puncture, with attention to opening pressure, cerebrospinal fluid protein, and cell counts. Xanthochromia in the cerebrospinal fluid usually is seen 3–4 hours after bleeding. If CT head scan and lumbar puncture are negative, SAH is doubtful. If lumbar puncture or CT head scan is positive for bleeding, obtain a four-vessel cerebral angiogram.

Remember: An angiogram may not show an aneurysm (because of hematoma formation or vasospasm). In highly suspected cases, the angiogram should be repeated in 1–2 weeks. Complications of aneurysmal SAH are rebleeding, intracerebral hematoma, intraventricular hemorrhage, acute hydrocephalus, delayed ischemic stroke caused by vasospasm, seizure, hyponatremia, syndrome of inappropriate antidiuretic hormone, cardiac ischemia, and arrhythmia (caused by autonomic hyperactivity).

When **treating subarachnoid hemorrhage aneurysm**, do the following:

1. Grade the patient's clinical status.

2. Consult a neurosurgeon as soon as SAH is suspected.
3. Admit the patient to the intensive care ward, monitor vital signs and neurologic status, order complete bed rest, elevate the patient's head to 30 degrees, and start IV fluid with normal saline. Control BP and cardiac arrhythmia, correct hyponatremia, and administer prophylactic antiepileptic drugs. Control pain and headache; prescribe a stool softener; treat vasospasm (important to recognize) with nimodipine, 60 mg taken orally every 6 hours; and hydrate with IV fluid.

Surgical treatments can include evacuation of the hematoma, insertion of a ventriculoperitoneal shunt (acute hydrocephalus), and clipping the aneurysm to prevent rebleed. Most authorities recommend early clipping of the aneurysm in patients with mild neurologic dysfunction (grades 1 and 2).

STROKE CAUSED BY DISSECTION OF EXTRACRANIAL ARTERIES

- Dissection of extracranial arteries is recognized increasingly as a cause of stroke in young adults.
- Dissection of arteries is caused by trauma in approximately 50% of cases and frequently from trivial trauma to the neck, such as a head turn, or neck twist.

- Carotid and vertebral arteries are frequent sites of dissection.
- Dissection-induced stroke is caused by acute arterial stenosis or embolization at the top of the dissection or aneurysm formation.
- Carotid dissection presents with neck or retro-orbital pain, followed by focal neurologic signs and symptoms. Check for carotid bruits and Horner's syndrome on the same side of the neck or eye pain.
- Diagnosis of dissection is established by cerebral angiography, but carotid Doppler ultrasonography, MRI, and magnetic resonance angiography may provide useful information.
- Most authorities recommend anticoagulation (heparin and warfarin) if hemorrhagic stroke or large stroke does not exist. Anticoagulation may continue for 3 months, followed by a repeat cerebral angiogram to assess opening of the artery and recanalization.

ISOLATED CENTRAL NERVOUS SYSTEM VASCULITIS

- Isolated CNS vasculitis or angiitis affects small arteries and capillaries of the brain and spinal cord without systemic involvement.
- CNS vasculitis is an immune-mediated condition, although sometimes it is seen after drug abuse (cocaine).

- Clinical features include headache, mental confusion (encephalopathy), multifocal neurologic signs, and seizure.
- Sedimentation rate is either normal or mildly elevated. Cerebrospinal fluid may show increased protein concentration and mild lymphocytic pleocytosis.
- Diagnosis is supported by cerebral angiography, which shows beading. However, an angiogram may be negative and lacks specificity because beading may be seen in nonvasculitic conditions such as infectious process, atherosclerosis, and neoplastic angioendotheliosis. In cases highly suspected for CNS vasculitis, cortical brain and leptomeningeal biopsy are warranted. Brain biopsy may be hampered by sampling error (sensitivity is approximately 80–85%).
- After a diagnosis of CNS vasculitis is established, the patient should be treated promptly with a high dose of prednisone and cyclophosphamide, with cyclophosphamide continuing for at least a year. Some authorities recommend repeating an angiogram before stopping cyclophosphamide.

COMMON CLINICAL STROKE SCENARIOS

Causes of Stroke in Young Adults

- Dissection of extracranial vessels of carotid (carotid and vertebral)

- Cardiogenic embolization
- CNS vasculitis
- Arthrosclerosis
- Drugs (cocaine, phenylpropanolamine)
- Moyamoya disease
- Coagulopathy (protein C and S deficiencies, antithrombin III deficiency, antiphospholipid antibody syndrome)
- Sickle cell anemia
- Cerebral venous thrombosis

Anterior Circulation Transient Ischemic Attacks and Stroke

Anterior circulation consists of the internal carotid artery and its branches: the middle cerebral artery, the anterior cerebral artery, and the penetrating branches of the middle cerebral artery and anterior cerebral artery (lenticulostriate). Anterior circulation TIAs and stroke present with lateralizing signs (motor and sensory), speech difficulties, ipsilateral cranial nerve dysfunction, and occasional contralateral vision loss (amaurosis fugax).

Posterior Circulation Transient Ischemic Attacks and Stroke

Posterior circulation consists of the vertebrobasilar arteries and their branches, posterior cerebral arteries, penetrating branches (paramedians), and thalamoperforates. Posterior circulation TIAs and stroke present with diffuse

neurologic symptoms and signs referable to the brain
stem and cerebellum, including dizziness, bilateral
blurred vision, diplopia, ataxia, multiple cranial nerve
dysfunction, and unilateral or bilateral motor and sensory
deficit. Isolated signs or symptoms rarely are related to
posterior circulation ischemic events.

Use of Anticoagulation in Stroke

Anticoagulates are given to stroke patients to prevent
further stroke or TIAs and to prevent potentially devas-
tating neurologic deficit (locked-in syndrome or coma, as
in basilar artery thrombosis). Although scientifically
unproven, anticoagulate therapy is indicated in the following stroke conditions:

- Noninfectious cardiogenic embolic stroke or TIAs
- Basilar artery thrombosis
- Series of TIAs (crescendo TIAs)
- Dissection of extracranial vessels

Following is a description of how anticoagulants
should be used:

- Establish an indication.
- Obtain a noncontrast CT scan of the head; repeat the
  scan in 24–48 hours if symptoms worsen.
- If head CT scan shows small ischemic stroke, initiate
  anticoagulation.

- If head CT scan shows large ischemic stroke with edema or hemorrhage, then wait 2–3 weeks. After that time, repeat CT scan. If hemorrhage or edema is resolving, then initiate anticoagulation.
- Control the patient's BP before administering anticoagulant if the patient is severely hypertensive.
- Begin anticoagulant with continuous infusion of heparin, then switch to warfarin, maintaining international normalized ratio to 2.0–2.5 of control. Many clinical conditions require temporary (weeks to months) anticoagulant therapy. Cardiogenic embolic events usually require chronic anticoagulation.

Aphasia

Aphasia, usually caused by stroke, is an acquired language disorder. The patient should be awake, alert, and able to hear before aphasia is assessed. Bedside testing for 5–10 minutes can establish which of the four common aphasias—expressive, global, receptive, or conduction—is present:

- Establish the **spontaneous (spoken) language** and determine if it is fluent or nonfluent.
- **Check the patient's ability to repeat a phrase.**
- **Check** the patient's **comprehension**.

A patient with **nonfluent** spontaneous speech and poor repetition and comprehension skills is affected with **global** aphasia. A patient with **nonfluent** speech and poor repetition skill but relatively good comprehension skill is affected with expressive Broca's aphasia (motor or anterior aphasia).

Remember: Most nonfluent aphasias are global. Nonfluent aphasia usually is associated with contralateral motor paresis and visual field defect. These patients are unable to write with either hand. A patient with **fluent** spontaneous speech but difficulty with repetition and comprehension has **receptive**, Wernicke's, posterior, or sensory aphasia. A patient with **fluent** speech but poor repetition skill and relatively good comprehension has **conduction** aphasia.

Caveat: All patients with these common aphasias have poor repetition skills, and the lesion involves the perisylvian region of the dominant hemisphere (**language zone**), which is supplied by the **middle cerebral artery**. A patient who has difficulty reading (alexia) with or without difficulty writing (agraphia) has a lesion in the **posterior cerebral artery** distribution.

9

Seizure and Epilepsy

- Seizures are transient, abnormal, massive neuronal discharges of the cerebral cortex that result in abnormal stereotyped behavior and represent a manifestation or symptom of a number of medical conditions. Epilepsy is defined as the occurrence of two or more unprovoked seizures. Epilepsy is a chronic disorder and, like seizure, is caused by many medical and neurologic conditions.
- Approximately 10% of individuals reaching age 70 years will have one seizure during their lifetime, but only 1–2% become epileptic.
- Seizure should be differentiated from syncope, migraine, transient ischemic attacks, multiple sclerosis, hypoglycemic attack, sleep disorders (narcolepsy, cataplexy, night terror), anxiety attacks, and pseudoseizure.
- Routine workup for the onset of unprovoked seizure in adults includes complete blood cell count, chemistry profile, electroencephalography (EEG), and magnetic resonance imaging (MRI). Further workup depends on individual conditions.
- The most important component in evaluating patients with first-time seizure is a good history. The seizure

event and postictal symptoms and signs are especially important.

- EEG is a gold standard test for diagnosing seizure and epilepsy; however, EEGs obtained between seizures (interictal) are positive in only 50% of patients with partial epilepsies and positive in approximately 60–65% in patients with generalized epilepsy. Therefore, normal EEGs do not rule out the diagnosis of epilepsy. An EEG recorded during a seizure is called *ictal*; an EEG obtained immediately after a seizure is called *postictal*.
- Most adult seizures can be classified as **partial (focal)**, **generalized**, or **partial seizure secondarily generalized**.
- Partial seizures originate from a discrete area of the brain, and an EEG shows focal spikes and sharp wakes. Partial seizures are classified further into simple partial seizures and complex partial seizures.
  - **Simple partial seizures** are characterized by the following manifestation types: motor, sensory, somatosensory, and psychic.
  - **Complex partial seizures** originate in the following brain areas: temporal lobe, frontal lobe, parietal lobe, and occipital lobe.
  - The difference between simple and complex partial seizure is impairment of consciousness, which occurs in complex partial seizure. Aura is a simple partial seizure.

- Generalized seizures arise from bilateral diffuse hemispheres. An EEG shows generalized, bilateral spike and wave discharges.
- Generalized seizures with onset in adulthood include
  - **Primary generalized seizures** (absence [petit mal], generalized tonic-clonic [grand mal], myoclonic)
  - **Secondary generalized with partial onset**
- Mistaking absence seizures for complex partial seizures not only leads to inappropriate workup, but also to incorrect therapy. Complex partial seizures last longer (30 seconds to 2–3 minutes) and may be preceded by an aura, and postictally the patient is confused, disoriented, and amnestic.
- Knowledge of seizure classifications helps clinicians plan a workup, choose the right drug therapy, suspect etiology, and prognosticate. Diagnosis of epilepsy should be firmly established before treatment begins.
- Patients with intractable seizure should be re-evaluated by MRI, which may show a new lesion, and a repeated EEG, which may show a change in seizure type. These patients should be referred to an epilepsy center for possible surgical intervention or antiepileptic drug (AED) trial studies. The most common form of surgery for treatment of intractable seizure is temporal lobectomy. Another surgical option is corpus callosotomy (disconnection), performed for intractable generalized seizure.

- Drug therapy goals in epilepsy are to prevent seizures and improve the patient's quality of life with the fewest side effects. Starting an AED is simple; the discontinuation is difficult. The patient's family should be involved in the care for epilepsy. Discuss drug reactions and side effects with the patient and the patient's family.
- Prescribe an AED based on seizure type. Always start with only one medication (monotherapy). Some patients later may need polypharmacy (e.g., status epilepticus, multiple seizure type) rather than monotherapy. The frequency of drug administration depends on its half-life (a shorter half-life equals more frequent dosing). Unless the patient has frequent seizures, start with a low dose of an AED and increase slowly. Check the drug level when the level reaches a steady state (usually $5 \times$ drug half-life). When seizures are controlled with subtherapeutic AED doses, increases are not necessary. The drug level should not be checked routinely at each visit. The level should be used as a guide when there is concern about compliance, drug toxicity, or drug interaction. When dose reaches a steady stage, increase it slowly (e.g., increase phenytoin by 30 mg); a full-dose increase (100 mg) may result in overdose. In seizure breakthrough, find the precipitating factors before dosage increase or change or addition of another AED.
- Sedative AEDs, such as phenobarbital or primidone, are not recommended for adult patients.

- In **status epilepticus**, prescribe a drug that can be given intravenously, acts quickly, reaches the brain rapidly, has a longer half-life, and causes less sedation.
- Several new AEDs are on the market. Before prescribing them, know their indications and side effects. Patients who do not respond to conventional AEDs should be referred to a neurologist.
- Establish the seizure control, quality of life, and drug side effects in follow-up appointments. Limited neurologic examination should include cognition and cerebellar function. Blood work, AED level, or other testing should not be repeated routinely and should be individualized according to type of seizure, symptoms, and signs. For asymptomatic patients, twice-a-year blood work (complete blood cell count and chemistry profile) is sufficient. Mentally retarded patients may need more frequent blood work.
- Most neurologists do not treat single, unprovoked, generalized tonic-clonic seizure, particularly if the patient's EEG, neuroimaging, and neurologic examination show normal results. Treatment for a single seizure should be considered if a recurrent seizure can be serious (e.g., truck drivers, workers at high-risk jobs). The chance of recurrence after a single seizure is approximately 20–25%.
- Do not change AED therapy during pregnancy; if necessary, do so before or after pregnancy. Avoid polypharmacy in pregnant women. Pregnant epileptic patients

should be seen monthly in the clinic and the AED should be checked. Do not use valproate in pregnancy. If a pregnant woman is taking valproate or carbamazepine, check her alpha-fetoprotein level and conduct an ultrasound during the first trimester, as the chance of fetal malformation in pregnant epileptic patients is three to four times greater than in nonepileptic women. There is no contraindication for epileptic mothers to breast feed.

- Head trauma is probably the most frequent preventable cause of epilepsy in industrial countries.
- Epileptic patients are permitted to drive motor vehicles, but each state and country has its own laws and regulations. As a clinician, you should know the laws in the state where you practice. Some states require a physician's report concerning epileptics. Statistically, epileptics do not have a higher motor vehicle accident rate than nonepileptics.
- Typical alcohol withdrawal seizures do not require maintenance AED therapy.
- Consider pseudoseizure when patients report recurrent seizures despite trial of several AEDs. Although there are many ways to differentiate true seizure from pseudoseizure, the definite diagnosis often needs prolonged video and EEG monitoring. Pseudoseizures often occur in association with true seizures.
- Onset of epilepsy in elderly patients should be evaluated by EEG and MRI head scan. AEDs that cause no signifi-

cant sedation or drug interaction should be administered in low dosage and gradually increased. Elderly patients often take several medications. Check for interactions.

- Epileptic patients do not necessarily remain epileptic for life. Patients with absence seizure may outgrow seizures. AED therapy discontinuation is a possibility in children when the patient is seizure-free for 2–3 years. Most neurologists do not discontinue AEDs in patients with partial seizures, mental retardation, or multiple seizure types. Patients with juvenile myoclonic epilepsy should continue medication for life.
- AED withdrawal should be considered under the following circumstances:
  - The patient has childhood-onset epilepsy.
  - Seizures are of generalized type, particularly primary generalized.
  - EEG, neuroimaging, and neurologic examination are normal.
  - The patient is seizure-free for 2–3 years.
  - The patient has history of infrequent seizures.
- When discontinuing AED therapy, take the following precautions:
  - Discuss with the patient and family the risks and benefits of stopping AED. Document the discussion in the chart and obtain the patient's written consent.
  - Obtain an EEG and AED level.
  - If the patient takes more than one AED, taper off one drug at a time.

- Discontinue medication slowly over 6–12 months.
- Advise the patient not to drive or work in high-risk jobs, and to avoid sleep deprivation and alcohol consumption during the withdrawal period.
- If seizures recur, reinstitute the medication and continue it for an indefinite time.
- New AEDs include the following:
  - Felbamate (Felbatol; introduced in 1993) requires frequent laboratory monitoring (blood count and liver function test). Felbamate is indicated in patients with refractory seizure, particularly patients with Lennox-Gastaut syndrome.
  - Gabapentin (Neurontin; mechanism action is unknown) is eliminated from the kidney and has no drug interaction. It may be the drug of choice for seizures in acute intermittent porphyria. The effective dose is 3,600–4,800 mg in divided doses, to be begun with lower dose. Gabapentin is effective in patients with partial and secondarily generalized seizure.
  - Lamotrigine (Lamictal; released in 1995) possibly blocks the sodium channel. It is effective against absence, generalized tonic clonic, and secondarily generalized seizures. It is also effective in Lennox-Gastaut syndrome. The most common side effects are dizziness, diplopia, and ataxia. Approximately 10% of patients report skin rash, particularly in children, if the patient takes valproate, or if dose is increased faster. Slow titration is recommended.

- Topiramate (Topamax; released in 1997) is effective against partial and generalized seizures in adults and children. The most common side effects are sedation and weight loss. Kidney stones occur in approximately 15% of patients. Slow titration is recommended. Recommended dosage is 25–50 mg per day with a weekly increase of up to 200–400 mg per day.
- Tiagabine (Gabitril; approved in October 1997) is effective against partial and secondarily generalized seizures. The average dosage in adults is 32–64 mg per day with slow titration.
- Vigabatrin (Sabril) and oxcarbazepine are not yet released in the United States.
- Most new AEDs are currently used as adjunctive therapy.

10

Central Nervous System Infections

CLINICAL TIPS

- Suspect central nervous system (CNS) infection in patients with fever, headache, nausea, vomiting, photophobia, altered mental state, or focal neurologic deficit.
- The triad of symptoms in meningitis includes fever, headaches, and neck stiffness, although these symptoms may be absent in the elderly and newborn.
- Encephalitis is indicated when behavior and personality changes, mental dysfunction, and seizure with or without focal neurologic deficit are observed.
- Meningitis and encephalitis often appear together (meningoencephalitis).
- All patients with CNS infection should have cultures, brain neuroimaging (computed tomography scan, magnetic resonance imaging [MRI]), and cerebrospinal fluid (CSF) examination.
- Begin empiric broad-spectrum antibiotic and acyclovir as soon as CNS infection is suspected.

- Consult an infectious disease specialist when CNS infection is indicated.

MENINGITIS

Bacterial Meningitis

- Bacterial meningitis is a medical emergency (see Chapter 25 for a discussion of acute meningitis).
- In suspected cases, promptly obtain a blood culture (which can be positive in 40% of patients with meningitis) and begin a combination of broad-spectrum antibiotics. The choice of antibiotic is simply an educated guess based on the age of the patient and underlying risk factors. One of the following combinations is recommended for adults:
  - Ceftriaxone (8–12 g/day) combined with vancomycin (2 g/day), administered four times a day intravenously (IV)
  - Ceftriaxone and ampicillin
  - Ceftriaxone and chloramphenicol
- In pneumococcal meningitis, CSF should be examined 48 hours after antimicrobial therapy and 48 hours after the treatment course, which usually lasts 2 weeks.
- The two leading pathogens of bacterial meningitis in adults are *Streptococcus pneumoniae* (pneumococcus) and *Neisseria meningitidis*. Risk factors for developing bacterial meningitis are immunosuppression (as in acquired immunodeficiency syndrome [AIDS] or caused

by immunosuppressive drugs), alcoholism, IV drug abuse, congenital heart disease, sinusitis, cancer, basilar skull fracture, sepsis, pneumonia, and sickle cell anemia.

- Recurrent bacterial meningitis (often caused by pneumococcus) is seen in patients with basilar skull fracture (which allows CSF leak), sinusitis, sickle cell anemia, and splenectomy. Meningitis may also be caused by ventriculoperitoneal shunt or intracranial surgery used to treat head trauma; in these cases, the infection is usually caused by *Staphylococcus aureus*.

- Complications of bacterial meningitis include increased intracranial pressure, cerebral edema, brain abscess, cortical venous thrombosis, epilepsy, subepidural and epidural abscess, hydrocephalus, mental retardation, hearing loss, and syndrome of inappropriate secretion of antidiuretic hormone.

- A persistent fever or predominantly neutrophilic pleocytosis signifies inadequate or wrong combination of antibiotic therapy, a resistant pathogen, a parameningeal infection source, or a brain abscess.

Viral (Aseptic) Meningitis

- Viral meningitis presents with low-grade fever, headache, malaise, and neck stiffness or tenderness. CSF examination usually reveals predominantly lymphocytic pleocytosis, mild elevation of protein concentration, and normal cultures. Treatment is supportive.

- When herpes simplex encephalitis is suspected, perform brain imaging and electroencephalography (EEG) and send blood and CSF for herpes simplex virus antibody and DNA (polymerase chain reaction [PCR]) testing. Begin acyclovir therapy (10 mg/kg IV q8h for 2–3 weeks).

Tuberculous Meningitis

- The incidence of tuberculous (TB) meningitis is increasing.
- The results of purified protein derivative testing and chest x-ray can be negative.
- PCR testing frequently is used because it provides faster results.
- Treatment of TB meningitis consists of four drug therapies:
  - Isoniazid (5 mg/kg/day orally)
  - Rifampin (600 mg/day orally)
  - Pyrazinamide (15–30 mg/kg/day orally)
  - Ethambutol (15–25 mg/kg/day orally)
- The combination therapy should continue for 2 months, until sensitivity is known, then decreased to two drugs. Drug therapy should continue for 1 year, and lumbar punctures should be performed periodically.

NEUROSYPHILIS

- Positive serology for syphilis (e.g., fluorescent treponemal antibody absorption test) in a patient with an unclear history of partial treatment indicates the need for lumbar puncture.
- Active neurosyphilis is usually associated with increased levels of white blood cells, protein, and immunoglobulin M and increased VDRL titer in the CSF.

Clinical Syndromes

- **Asymptomatic** (common clinical scenario in which CSF is abnormal but there are no neurologic deficits or signs)
- **Meningovascular**
- **Tabes** (loss of proprioception, painless foot ulcers, joint destruction [Charcot joint], abnormal pupillary reaction [Argyll-Robertson], sensory ataxia, and lightning pain)
- **General paresis** (slowly progressive, personality changes, dementia, myoclonic jerks, seizure, and focal neurologic deficits)

Treatment

Treatment of neurosyphilis includes aqueous penicillin G, 2–4 million units q4h IV for 10 days, followed by 2.4 million units of benzathine penicillin administered intramuscularly once a week for 3 weeks. If the patient is allergic

to penicillin, substitute tetracycline or chloramphenicol
for 1 month.

CREUTZFELDT-JAKOB DISEASE

- Creutzfeldt-Jakob disease (CJD), or spongiform
  encephalopathy, is a transmissible disorder related
  to bovine spongiform encephalopathy, or "mad cow
  disease."
- The causative agent is prion, a protein without DNA.
- CJD presents with rapidly progressive dementia,
  myoclonic jerks, ataxia, and upper and lower motor
  neuron signs.
- When the disease is established, an EEG commonly
  shows periodic 1- to 2-Hz, generalized sharp, triphasic
  waves.
- The diagnosis is made by brain biopsy or at autopsy.
- Because CJD is transmissible, deceased demented
  patients should not be used for organ donation.

ACQUIRED IMMUNODEFICIENCY SYNDROME

- Neurologic symptoms and signs indicate the onset of
  AIDS in 10–13% of cases.
- Approximately 50% of patients with positive human
  immunodeficiency virus (HIV) antibody tests develop
  a neurologic disorder during the course of illness, and

as many as 95% of patients with AIDS have neuropathologic changes in the nervous system at autopsy.
- Neurologic complications generally correlate with level of CD4 count in the blood (a lower CD4 count is associated with more severe neurologic problems).

Neurologic Complications

- Neurologic complications of AIDS appear in the central and peripheral nervous systems.
- In the **CNS**, direct effects of retrovirus (HIV) include
  - Subacute and chronic meningitis
  - AIDS encephalopathy (dementia)
  - Myelopathy
- Indirect effects of HIV include
  - Opportunistic infections
  - Stroke
  - Lymphoma
- In the **peripheral nervous system (PNS)**, change to the following HIV-associated neuropathies:
  - Acute demyelinating polyneuropathy (Guillain-Barré syndrome)
  - Chronic inflammatory demyelinating polyneuropathy
  - Mononeuritis multiplex
  - Distal, symmetric, sensory painful neuropathy
  - Cytomegalovirus radiculopathy
- The following HIV-associated myopathies:

- Inflammatory myopathy (polymyositis)
- Nemaline or rodlike myopathy
- Drug-induced neuromyopathy in the PNS include
  - Distal, sensory, and painful neuropathy caused by zidovudine (AZT), 2'3'dideoxyinosine, 2'3'-dideoxy-cytidine, or stavudine.
  - Mitochondrial myopathy caused by AZT presents with proximal weakness, myalgia, and elevated serum creatine kinase.

AIDS Encephalopathy

AIDS encephalopathy, or dementia, presents with apathy, personality changes, tremor, myoclonia, seizure, ataxia, dementia, bradykinesia, and long-tract signs. Diagnosis is supported by MRI of the brain, which shows diffuse atrophy. CSF examination shows elevation of protein concentration and level of β_2-microglobulin (normal is <3.8 mg/liter) and positive PCR testing.

AIDS Myelopathy

AIDS myelopathy occurs in 10–15% of patients with AIDS. It presents with proprioception loss, spastic paraparesis, and incontinence (similar to subacute combined degeneration of the cord caused by vitamin B_{12} deficiency).

11

Alteration of Mental Status

Alteration of mental status is a common cause of hospital admission, and neurologists are often asked to evaluate these patients in consultation.

WHAT YOU SHOULD ESTABLISH WHEN EVALUATING PATIENTS WITH ALTERATION OF MENTAL STATUS

- Onset of illness (acute, subacute, or chronic)
- Course (rapidly progressive, nonprogressive, slowly progressive, or fluctuating)
- Underlying medical diseases
- Pre-existing primary neurologic problems (e.g., seizure, stroke, or dementia)
- Use of medication that may affect mental function, recent change in medication dosage, or addition of new drug to the patient's regimen

DELIRIUM

Delirium is simply an **acute confusion state**. The hallmarks are disorientation, inattentiveness, and global impairment of cognitive function. Although in practice delirium is known to be associated with autonomic over-activity such as fever, tachycardia, hallucination, and tremor, the lethargic form of delirium is more common. Therefore one of the clinical characteristics of delirium is a fluctuating state of alertness.

What You Should Do

1. Take a detailed medical, psychological, and neuro-logic history (often obtained indirectly through family members).
2. Perform a general physical examination (to assess underlying medical cause) and neurologic examination (to assess particularly whether organic brain disease or a focal brain lesion exists; be aware that it is easy to miss a subdural hematoma in a delirious patient). Pay special attention to cognitive function; pupillary size, symmetry, and reactivity; whether the neck is stiff; and the motor examination and the presence of any involuntary movements (e.g., tremor, myoclonia, chorea, or asterixis).
3. **Try to identify the underlying cause (or causes):**
   - **Toxic and metabolic encephalopathies** are the most common causes of delirium. *Encephalopathy* is a nonspecific term for global confusion caused by diffuse brain dysfunction. Metabolic conditions causing encephalopathy include electrolyte

imbalance; renal, hepatic, or pulmonary failure; endocrine disorders; and septicemia. Many environmental toxins can produce encephalopathy, but drug-induced encephalopathy is more common. Remember that adding new drugs or a minor change in the drug regimen of an elderly patient may cause delirium. Drugs known to cause confusion include anticholinergics, antihistamines, antihypertensives, digitalis, antipsychotics, antiparkinsonian agents, steroids, antidepressants, cocaine, lysergic acid diethylamide (LSD), and alcohol.

- **Multifocal brain lesions**, as in patients with meningoencephalitis, vasculitis, or acquired immunodeficiency syndrome, may cause delirium.
- A **focal brain lesion**, as in right parietal stroke, or a lesion involving the limbic system or memory regions can also manifest as mental confusion.

Hints for Assessing Delirium

Acute mental confusion in an elderly patient with no evidence of a focal brain lesion is most likely due to an underlying infection (urologic in women), drug regimen changes, or hypoxia. In a young patient with a similar presentation, drug overdose or drug or alcohol withdrawal are the most likely causes.

DEMENTIA

What You Should Know

- Dementia is an acquired brain disorder characterized by a decline of cognitive and intellectual function, leading to mental, physical, and social disability, and dependency. Before considering the diagnosis of dementia, you should establish that the patient has intact sensorium (i.e., is alert and awake); sensorium is impaired in delirium.
- Dementia should be suspected when the patient
  - Gets confused by minor distraction
  - Exhibits slowness of movements
  - Exhibits emotional lability or irritability
  - Gets lost
  - Misuses words
- Dementia should be distinguished from the following conditions in which the patient appears to be demented: senile forgetfulness, depression (pseudo-dementia), psychiatric illness (schizophrenia), aphasia, transient global amnesia, or nonconvulsive (absence or complex partial) status epilepticus.
- Approximately 4% of people older than age 65 and 20% older than age 85 are demented. Only 10% of the causes of dementia are reversible; therefore, full evaluation in all demented patients is necessary.

Causes of Dementia

The causes of dementia are generally either medical, neuro-logic, or psychiatric. In the elderly population, Alzheimer's disease (AD) is the leading cause (50–75%). Vascular dementias and Parkinson's disease (PD) are the other leading causes. Dementia may also be caused by diffuse Lewy bodies, depression, toxic and metabolic disorders, infections, structural lesions, and alcohol.

Alzheimer's Disease
Diagnosis
The probable diagnosis of AD can be made when a patient has the following symptoms and other causes have been excluded:

- Slowly progressive dementia
- Prominent, progressive memory loss and at least one other cognitive dysfunction
- Onset after age 60
- No focal deficit or gait problem at the onset

The definite diagnosis of AD may only be made by brain biopsy or at autopsy.

Treatment
The caregivers of AD should be educated about the disease and provided with sources of social support and community resources.

DEPRESSION

Depression occurs in 30–50% of patients with AD. Selective serotonin reuptake inhibitors have fewer side effects than conventional tricyclic antidepressants. Paroxetine (Paxil), 10–40 mg per day, and sertraline (Zoloft), 25–100 mg per day, are the drugs of choice. If a tricyclic antidepressant is indicated, nortriptyline (Pamelor), 10–75 mg per day, is recommended.

SLEEP DISORDERS

Sleep disorders are common in patients with AD, particularly in nursing home patients. Trazodone (Desyrel), 25–100 mg at night, is recommended.

COGNITION

Two medications, both cholinergics, have been approved for improving cognition in patients with AD: tacrine (Cognex) and donepezil (Aricept). Tacrine requires tight titration, and the response is dose dependent (120–160 mg/day). Liver function should be monitored carefully every 2 weeks for the first 18 weeks of therapy. Aricept is easier to use (5–10 mg/day) and has fewer side effects.

DISEASE PROGRESSION

Estrogen, nonsteroidal anti-inflammatory drugs, prednisone, vitamin E, and selegiline may slow the disease progression.

Vascular or Multi-Infarct Dementia

Vascular or multi-infarct dementia is suspected when a patient has

- Clear mental impairment after stroke
- A fluctuating course with stepwise worsening
- Unilateral or bilateral corticospinal tract findings
- Pseudobulbar features
- Strong risk factors for stroke

Dementia with Lewy Bodies

Dementia with Lewy bodies is characterized by the following:

- Progressive dementia
- Early parkinsonism without tremor
- Fluctuating confusion, hallucinosis
- REM behavioral disorder
- Increased neuroleptic sensitivity

Parkinsonian Features and Dementia

Parkinsonian features and dementia are seen in

- Primary PD (dementia occurs in 40%)
- Late-stage AD
- Progressive supranuclear palsy
- Diffuse Lewy body disease
- Primary nigral degeneration
- Corticobasal degeneration

What You Should Do in Evaluating a Demented Patient

1. Obtain a detailed history (medical, neurologic, and psychiatric) from the patient, relatives, and care-givers and try to establish the onset and course of dementia.

2. Perform a detailed medical and neurologic examination. When performing the neurologic examination, pay special attention to **cognitive function**; generally, the Mini-Mental State Examination (MMSE) is sufficient.

    Caveat: When performing the MMSE, try not to irritate the patient, and explain the purpose of your questions. The patient's level of education and age and whether he or she is taking sedative medication will affect the test results. Well-educated patients can perform well even when their cognition is impaired. In these patients, formal neuropsychological testing is necessary.

3. Establish whether there is a focal neurologic deficit and whether the patient has a prominent gait or motor problem.

4. Observe for any involuntary movements such as chorea, myoclonus, and tremor dystonia.

5. Look for the following signs, which are commonly found in demented patients:
    • Grasp, rooting, snout, and palmomental reflex

- Glabellar sign (seen in patients with PD)
- Increased jaw jerk
- Paratonia (gegenhalten, or resistance to all passive movements of the joints)
- Motor perseveration (repeating a motor task)
- Motor impersistence (inability to maintain a motor task such as keeping eyes closed, keeping tongue out, or maintaining hand grip)

Workup

The following tests are recommended in all demented patients: complete blood cell count, chemistry profile, chest x-ray, electrocardiogram, thyroid function tests (thyroxine, thyroid-stimulating hormone), vitamin B_{12} and folate level measurement, syphilis serology, and head neuroimaging. The following tests are considered for selected patients with dementia: electroencephalogram, lumbar puncture, human immunodeficiency virus testing, heavy metal screen, positron emission tomography (PET) or single photon emission computed tomography (SPECT) scan, angiogram, neuropsychometric testing, or brain biopsy.

Some Points about Workup

- It is not uncommon to find low vitamin B_{12} levels in the elderly; thus, a significant deficiency should be further confirmed by determination of serum methylmalonic acid and homocysteine levels or a trial of vitamin B_{12} therapy.

- Electroencephalography is recommended when the clinical presentation suggests a seizure disorder or Creutzfeldt-Jakob disease.
- Computed tomography or magnetic resonance imaging is particularly useful when
  - The patient has had symptoms of dementia for less than 6 months
  - The onset occurred when the patient was younger than 60 years
  - The patient has a history of seizures
  - The patient has focal neurologic signs
  - The patient has gait abnormalities
- Lumbar puncture is indicated when
  - The patient has experienced rapidly progressive dementia for less than 1 month
  - Chronic infection is suspected as a cause
  - The serum fluorescent treponemal antibody absorption test is positive
  - Normal-pressure hydrocephalus is suspected
  - The onset of dementia occurred when the patient was younger than 50 years
  - CNS vasculitis or meningeal carcinomatous lesion is suspected
- SPECT or PET can be useful in differentiating AD from vascular dementia.
- Routine genetic testing for AD is not indicated. No genetic test can accurately predict at what age an individual might be affected by the disease. If a family requests genetic testing, they should be referred to Alzheimer's Association (800-272-3900).

12

Demyelinating Disorders

Demyelinating disorders commonly seen in adults include the following:

- Multiple sclerosis (MS)
- Acute disseminated encephalomyelitis (ADEM)
- Acute transverse myelitis (ATM)
- Progressive multifocal leukoencephalopathy (PML)
- Cerebral pontine myelinolysis
- Acute optic neuritis (ON)

MULTIPLE SCLEROSIS

MS is the most common demyelinating disorder in young adults and probably is the leading cause of disability in the same age group. The disease affects the central nervous system (CNS) myelin, producing a "plaque." MS plaques characteristically are disseminated in the CNS, separated in time and space. The disease most commonly affects young women between the ages of 20 and 40 and has a higher prevalence in the northern United States than in other parts of the country. Most authorities believe it is an autoimmune disease that is triggered by viral or environmental factors in genetically predisposed individuals.

Clinical Course

- In 20% of patients with MS, the disease has a benign clinical course.
- In 30%, the disease is relapsing and remitting.
- In 50%, the disease is primarily progressive and secondarily progressive with relapse.

Initial Clinical Presentations

The most common symptoms of MS are sensory complaints (e.g., numbness, paresthesia), weakness, clumsiness, visual symptoms, and sphincter disturbances. The onset of MS is variable and differs from patient to patient. Because the initial symptoms are often subjective and nonanatomic (i.e., multifocal), both overdiagnosis and underdiagnosis of MS are common in clinical practice.

Symptoms and Signs Suggesting Multiple Sclerosis

- Unilateral ON
- Bilateral internuclear ophthalmoplegia
- Multifocal corticospinal tract signs
- Intention tremor

- Early bladder dysfunction (frequency, urgency)
- Lhermitte's sign
- Uhthoff's phenomenon (worsening of symptoms and signs after exposure to heat or exertion)
- Facial myokymia (spontaneous, undulating movements of the facial muscles)
- Charcot's triad (intention tremor, nystagmus, scanning speech)

When to Doubt the Diagnosis of Multiple Sclerosis

- Dementia
- Aphasia
- Seizure
- Pain (except trigeminal neuralgia)
- Movement disorders

Diagnosis

Clinical History and Neurologic Examination

To make the diagnosis of MS, it is important to establish the following through clinical history and neurologic examination:

- Two attacks (neurologic symptoms or deficit) and clinical evidence of two separate white matter lesions

- Two attacks lasting more than 24 hours, clinical evidence of one attack, and paraclinical evidence of another lesion 1 month or sooner after the first lesion
- One attack, clinical evidence of one, paraclinical evidence of another, and abnormal cerebrospinal fluid (CSF)
- Multifocal neurologic deficits referable to the CNS white matter
- Multifocal neurologic symptoms and signs with relapse and remission and no explanation by another neurologic condition

Diagnostic Tests

Diagnostic tests are ordered to support the clinical impression of MS and/or exclude other possibilities.

Magnetic Resonance Imaging of the Brain

Abnormalities on magnetic resonance imaging (MRI) of the brain have been reported in as many as 90% of patients with clinically diagnosed MS. The most common characteristic seen on MRI is increased signal intensity in T2-weighted images, showing multiple plaques that are typically oval (Dawson's fingers) and greater than 6 mm in diameter in the periventricular regions and perpendicular to the lateral ventricles. Other common sites of plaques are the posterior fossa, brain stem, and corpus callosum. The plaques are typically at different stages, meaning some of them enhance with contrast material (e.g., gadolinium). Spinal cord MRI may show plaque; in such a case, it is important to differentiate progressive MS from slow-growing tumors.

   Caveat: Normal MRI of the brain, with history and neurologic findings consistent with MS, does not rule out MS. Likewise, abnormal MRI of the brain, without history and neurologic findings consistent with MS, cannot allow you to make the diagnosis of MS with certainty. Normal MRI of the brain without a convincing history and physical examination make the diagnosis of MS unlikely. The number of plaques shown by MRI does not always correlate with the severity of the disease but might correlate with prognosis.

Cerebrospinal Fluid
CSF abnormalities in MS include

- Mild elevation of CSF protein concentration and lymphocytes (<35/mm)
- Elevation of immunoglobulin G (IgG) with oligoclonal band (seen in 90% of patients with definite MS)
- Increased IgG index (normal = <0.7), which indicates breakdown in the blood-brain barrier
- Increased myelin basic protein (normal = <1.0 ng/liter), which indicates activity of the disease. However, this is a very nonspecific measure.

Evoked Potentials
When an MRI cannot be performed or is unavailable, multimodality evoked potentials (visual, brain stem, and

somatosensory) may be used to establish multifocal sites of the lesion in the CNS and optic nerve, which can prove dissemination in space and not time, unless a previously normal evoked potential changes to abnormal. In uncooperative patients and patients in whom MRI cannot be performed (e.g., due to pacemaker), measuring evoked potentials is an alternative. The sensitivity of evoked potential testing is high but its specificity is low.

Prognosis

- The **"one-third rule"** with regard to MS means that, generally speaking, one-third of patients do well, one-third become disabled but continue their daily living activities independently, and one-third become wheel-chair bound.
- **Kurtzke's 5-year rule** is that "absence of significant motor or cerebellar deficit at 5 years correlates with limited disability at 15 years."
- A **good prognosis** may be expected when onset of the disease occurs before the patient is age 40, the clinical course is relapsing and remitting in a female patient, the patient has sensory complaints at the onset and infrequent exacerbation, and the patient has mild abnormalities on MRI at diagnosis.

Therapy

Acute Exacerbation

The following steps are taken for a patient experiencing an acute exacerbation of MS:

- Methylprednisolone (Solu-Medrol) (may be given on an outpatient basis as well). Administer methylprednisolone intravenously at a rate of 1 g per 90 minutes in a 5% dextrose solution with monitoring of blood pressure and pulse. The total dose is 500–1,000 mg per day for 5 days, followed by 2–4 weeks of prednisone tapered orally. The **side effects** of this treatment include headaches, dizziness, and muscle cramps.
- Check blood chemistry and urine.
- Treat an infection first if it exists.

Caveat: In a known case of MS, before considering methylprednisolone, exclude or treat a urinary tract infection, fever from any kind of infection, or electrolyte imbalance, because these conditions exacerbate neurologic deficit (pseudorelapse).

Relapsing and Remitting Multiple Sclerosis

Three compounds have been approved by the U.S. Food and Drug Administration for treatment of **relapsing and remitting MS**:

- **Interferon B-Ib (Betaseron):** 8 million units (250 mg of protein) given qod subcutaneously
- **Interferon B-Ia (Avonex):** 6 million units (30 mg of protein) given intramuscularly once a week
- **Copolymer-1 (Copaxone):** 20 mg given daily subcutaneously

These three compounds are used less often in patients with the secondary progressive type of MS unless there are still prominent superimposed relapses. All three drugs are equally effective in reducing the relapsing rate by 30%, but only Avonex has been proved to slow disability and progression. Avonex and Betaseron have been shown on MRI to decrease accumulation of new lesions. All three are equally expensive (approximately $1,000 a month) and are given on a long-term basis. These drugs are generally prescribed to patients with frequent relapses, severe relapses, or very abnormal MRI. The choice of which one to use depends on patient preference and physician familiarity.

The most common undesirable side effect of interferons is a flulike syndrome with severe chills and profuse sweating. Copaxone is not associated with the flulike syndrome and requires no laboratory monitoring.

Symptoms

The following medications are used to treat the symptoms of MS:

1. Spasticity
   - Baclofen, 10 mg tid up to 80 mg per day
   - Benzodiazepines
   - Dantrolene (Dantrium): 75 mg per day
2. Tremor
   - Beta blockers
   - Clonazepam
   - Gabapentin (Neurontin)
3. Depression
   - Tricyclic antidepressants or selective serotonin reuptake inhibitors
4. Pain
   - Tricyclic antidepressants
   - Carbamazepine
   - Gabapentin
5. Fatigue (common complaint)
   - Amantadine: 100 mg bid or tid
   - Pemoline (Cylert): 18.75 mg bid
   - Fluoxetine
6. Bladder dysfunction
   - Oxybutynin (Ditropan), 5 mg tid
   - Propantheline (Pro-Banthine)

Rehabilitation

Rehabilitation in MS patients includes physical and occupational therapy.

ACUTE DISSEMINATED ENCEPHALOMYELITIS

- ADEM is an acute, monophasic encephalitis that occurs after a viral illness or vaccination (postinfectious or parainfectious).
- It is more common in children than in adults and is believed to be caused by an immune response triggered by an antigen (viral or vaccine).
- The prognosis for recovery is generally good; recovery is usually spontaneous.
- The neurologic manifestations of ADEM include headache, malaise, confusion, lethargy, seizures, and multifocal neurologic deficits.
- The **features that most distinguish ADEM from MS** are its **monophasic** course and the absence of true relapse.
- Although the CSF evaluation, MRI, and histopathology of ADEM and MS may be similar, in ADEM the CSF IgG concentration is rarely elevated and oligoclonal bands are usually absent. CSF cell count in ADEM usually is greater than 50 lymphocytes per microliter.
- MRI of the brain typically shows multiple high signal intensity lesions involving white matter. The lesions usually are symmetric, and occipital head regions are predominantly involved. The lesions can affect gray matter and basal ganglia as well. In contrast to MS

plaques, the lesions are usually of the same age (i.e., they show more uniform enhancement).
- Treatment of ADEM is supportive and symptomatic, but many neurologists administer 5 days of pulse methylprednisolone treatment (1,000 mg/day).

ISOLATED IDIOPATHIC OPTIC NEURITIS

Clinical Features

Isolated idiopathic ON is characterized by the following:

- Acute onset of orbital pain, particularly eye pain on an eye movement test
- Central or paracentral scotoma
- Color desaturation
- Progressive, often unilateral vision loss

Examination

On examination a patient with isolated idiopathic ON will exhibit

- Decreased visual activity
- Impaired visual field
- Impaired color perception
- Afferent pupillary defect (Marcus Gunn pupil)
- Swollen disc with blurred margin (papillitis) or normal disc appearance (retrobulbar ON)

Relationship to Multiple Sclerosis

The risk of developing MS for a young adult with idio-pathic unilateral ON is approximately 30% after 10 years of follow-up. If the results of brain MRI are abnormal, the risk increases to 70–80% in 5 years. Most neurologists recommend MRI of the brain.

   Caveat: Not all patients with ON and abnormal MRI develop clinically definite MS.

Therapy

The natural history of ON is good; most cases resolve spontaneously. Intravenous methylprednisolone can speed the recovery but does not change the outcome at 6 months. Oral prednisone is no longer used because it can cause rebound flares of ON. Although its efficacy is scientifically unproven, most neurologists prescribe a course of pulse methylprednisolone treatment. Some authorities advocate steroid therapy for patients with abnormal MRI. The disease has a recurrence rate of 15–30%.

ACUTE TRANSVERSE MYELITIS

Clinical Features

The clinical features of ATM include

  • Acute flaccid paraparesis

- Sensory level deficit (commonly thoracic)
- Bowel or bladder dysfunction

The idiopathic form is rare.

Evaluation

Evaluation of the patient with suspected ATM includes the following tests: complete blood cell count, chemistry profile, rapid plasma reagin, erythrocyte sedimentation rate, vitamin B_{12} levels, human immunodeficiency virus (HIV), CSF, and MRI of the brain and spinal cord.

Relationship to Multiple Sclerosis

The risk of developing MS for a patient with idiopathic ATM and normal MRI is approximately 10%. If MRI of the brain is abnormal, the risk increases to 70%, and if the CSF is negative for bands, the risk of MS is very low.

Therapy

Therapy is supportive and symptomatic—intravenous pulse methylprednisolone when brain MRI is abnormal or the patient has a dense deficit. Prognosis is generally good, and complete recovery occurs in approximately two-thirds of patients.

PROGRESSIVE MULTIFOCAL LEUKOENCEPHALOPATHY

- PML is an opportunistic infection affecting the CNS myelin caused by reactivation of the JC virus and infection of oligodendrocytes in immunocompromised patients (e.g., due to acquired immunodeficiency syndrome, malignancy, or iatrogenic immunosuppression).
- As many as 7% of HIV-positive patients develop PML in the course of their illness.
- The clinical manifestations include progressive mental dysfunction, visual agnosia, seizures, incoordination, and multifocal neurologic deficits.
- MRI of the brain shows focal or multifocal increased signal intensity on T2-weighted images in the white matter (sometimes gray matter)with variable enhancement. CSF examination shows elevation of protein and mononuclear cells and abnormal JC virus on DNA analysis (polymerase chain reaction). Definite diagnosis is made by brain biopsy.
- Therapy is conservative. Intravenous zidovudine combined with intrathecal cytarabine (Ara-C) may be considered in some cases.

CENTRAL PONTINE MYELINOLYSIS

- Cerebral pontine myelinolysis is a rare demyelinating disease most commonly seen in alcoholics and malnourished patients.

- The cause is unknown but has been related to rapid correction of serum osmolality or hyponatremia.
- Clinical manifestations include lethargy, mental confusion, flaccid quadriparesis, and pseudobulbar palsy.
- Diagnosis is suspected when an alcoholic patient with hyponatremia becomes quadriparetic after correction of hyponatremia.
- MRI of the brain frequently shows a midline demyelinating lesion in the basis pons; the lesions also can be seen in the thalamus, basal ganglia, and subcortical white matter. There is no specific therapy, but slow correction of serum osmolality (12 mmol/liter/day) and hyponatremia (130–135 mmol/liter) will prevent the disease.

13

Neurologic Complications of Alcohol

Neurologic complications of alcohol include

1. Acute alcoholic intoxication, ranging from mild euphoria to coma (depending on the serum alcohol level)
2. Alcoholic blackout: transient amnesia after a binge
3. Alcohol withdrawal syndromes: tremulousness, autonomic hyperactivity, hallucinosis
4. Alcohol withdrawal seizures (see below)
5. Delirium tremens: confusion, florid hallucination, and autonomic hyperactivity
6. Nutritional deficiencies
   - Wernicke-Korsakoff syndrome
   - Alcoholic polyneuropathy
   - Pellagra
7. Neurologic complications of uncertain etiology
   - Alcoholic cerebellar degeneration
   - Central pontine myelinolysis
   - Marchiafava-Bignami syndrome (degeneration of corpus callosum)

- Alcoholic myopathy
- Alcoholic amblyopia
8. Encephalopathy
   - Hepatic encephalopathy
9. Trauma
   - Subdural hematoma
   - Post-traumatic epilepsy
10. Other neurologic association
    - Stroke
    - Movement disorders

ALCOHOL WITHDRAWAL SEIZURES

- Alcohol withdrawal seizures ("rum fits") occur approximately 24 hours after cessation or reduction of drinking after chronic use.
- The seizures are self-limited, brief, generalized tonic-clonic seizures and occur one to three in a row.
- Approximately 3% may present as status epilepticus.
- The majority of patients have other signs of withdrawal as well.
- Patients with uncomplicated cases have normal neurologic examination and brain imaging.
- Neuroimaging and electroencephalography (EEG) are warranted in patients with withdrawal seizures when they occur the first time and should be repeated thereafter if the patient's neurologic status has changed.

- EEG after seizure may show diffuse, nonspecific slowing; photomyoclonic response, however, may be seen.
- Alcohol withdrawal seizures do not lead to chronic epilepsy if the patient remains abstinent.
- Treatment includes hydration, administration of thiamine and benzodiazepines, and correcting low magnesium levels if they exist.
- Maintenance with chronic antiepileptic drugs (AEDs) usually is not required, because if the patient continues drinking, he or she still will have seizures and is unlikely to take medication, and if the patient stops drinking, he or she does not need AEDs. However, consider maintenance AEDs if
  - Seizures are focal
  - The patient has a focal neurologic deficit or focal structural insult demonstrated on brain imaging
  - The patient has epileptic discharges on EEG
- Status epilepticus in alcoholics must be treated like any other status epilepticus.

ALCOHOLIC NUTRITIONAL POLYNEUROPATHY

- Alcoholic nutritional polyneuropathy is a chronic, progressive, sensorimotor polyneuropathy that is predominantly axonal.

- The disease causes a painful, burning sensation in the feet and predominantly involves the lower extremities, causing depressed reflexes.
- Hyperhidrosis of the feet and hands is common.
- Treatment includes administration of thiamine and multivitamins and symptomatic treatment of pain.

ALCOHOLIC CEREBELLAR DEGENERATION

- Alcoholic cerebellar degeneration is a slowly progressive ataxia.
- Its typical features include impairment of stance and gait (truncal ataxia), with minimal or no nystagmus, dysarthria, or ataxia of the upper extremities.
- The pathology involves degeneration of the superior vermis (midline).
- It is often associated with a variable degree of polyneuropathy. Treatment is supportive and includes thiamine and multivitamins.

14

Dizziness and Vertigo

KEY POINTS OF THE HISTORY

Key points in taking a history from a patient with dizziness or vertigo include

- Differentiation of dizziness from true vertigo (sensation of movement) and other terms used by the patient
- Establishment of the onset of dizziness and whether it is acute, subacute, or chronic
- Aggravating factors, such as head or body position
- Associated symptoms, including those that suggest otologic etiologies (nausea, vomiting, fullness of ears, hearing loss, and tinnitus) and those that suggest central nervous system (CNS) etiologies (headaches, diplopia, blurred vision, ataxia, and paresthesia)
- History of recent ear or upper respiratory infection or head trauma
- History of drug regimen or drug overdose
- History of depression or other psychiatric problems

KEY POINTS OF PHYSICAL EXAMINATION

Key points of the physical examination of a patient with dizziness or vertigo include the following:

- Checking the cardiovascular system for cardiac arrhythmia, murmur, orthostatic hypotension, and carotid or subclavian bruits.
- Checking the ears for infection, trauma, or impacted wax.
- Performing a Nylen-Barany (Dix-Hallpike) test: Quickly move the patient from a sitting position on a table to lying down supine with the head positioned over the end of the table. Rotate the head 45 degrees side to side and observe for vertigo, nausea, and nystagmus (onset, direction, and duration). The presence of these symptoms or signs suggests vestibulopathy if they have delayed onset, are fatigable, and are unidirectional.
- Doing a complete neurologic examination with special attention to the brain stem, cranial nerves, and cerebellar function.

CAUSES OF VERTIGO

Vertigo is a multifactorial condition. The neurologist is often consulted to determine whether vertigo is caused by inner ear disease or a CNS lesion.

Central Nervous System Causes

- When vertigo is due to CNS causes, the onset may be acute, subacute, or chronic.
- When the head tilt test or Nylen-Barany test is performed, the onset of vertigo is sudden, without any latency or delay and does not fatigue (i.e., decrease severity with repetition of tilt).
- Nystagmus is often multidirectional, and nausea and vomiting, generalized fatigue, and hearing loss are less severe.
- Associated neurologic **symptoms and signs** (brain stem and cerebellar dysfunction) more strongly suggest CNS causes.
- **CNS causes of vertigo** include
  - Posterior circulation transient ischemic attack or stroke
  - Brain stem stroke or tumor
  - Cerebellopontine angle tumors
  - Posterior fossa pathologies
  - Multiple sclerosis
  - Spinocerebellar degeneration
  - Migraine variant

Drug-Induced Dizziness and Vertigo

The following medications may induce dizziness and vertigo:

- Aminoglycosides
- Penicillin
- Aspirin
- Sulfonamides
- Antiepileptic drugs
- Antihistamines

Common Otologic Causes of Vertigo

Benign Paroxysmal Positional Vertigo

- Benign paroxysmal positional vertigo is the most common cause of acute vertigo.
- It is thought to be caused by the presence of deposited otoconia (canalith) in the semicircular canal after head trauma or repeated ear infection.
- It is exacerbated by head or body movements or turning, particularly of the head.
- On the head-tilt test, the vertigo has delayed onset and is fatigable, and nystagmus is usually unidirectional.
- Hearing is intact and tinnitus rarely occurs.
- The caloric test is abnormal in approximately 50% of cases.
- Although it is generally self-limited, the condition is disabling at times.

Acute Labyrinthitis

- Acute labyrinthitis causes acute positional vertigo.

- It usually is proceeded by upper respiratory tract infection and may be associated with hearing loss.
- It is usually self-limited (5–7 days) but may result in permanent hearing loss.

Vestibular Neuronitis

- Vestibular neuronitis causes severe, acute vertigo associated with nausea and vomiting.
- The patient is apprehensive about moving and experiences fullness of the ear and tinnitus.
- It usually precedes a viral illness, and recovery may take 2–3 weeks.

EVALUATION OF A DIZZY PATIENT

Evaluation of a dizzy patient depends on the suspected cause after history and examination. If the patient has hearing loss and tinnitus and is suspected of having otologic disease, he or she should be evaluated by an ear, nose, and throat specialist for formal audiogram and caloric testing. If CNS causes are suspected, MRI of the head is indicated. A patient with dizziness of undetermined cause should be tested for complete blood cell count, erythrocyte sedimentation rate, chemistry profile, electrocardiogram, thyroid function, and fluorescent treponemal antibody.

SYMPTOMATIC DRUG THERAPY FOR DIZZINESS

Therapy for the symptoms of dizziness includes

- Anticholinergics: scopolamine disc (Transderm Scōp), 1.5 mg per disc behind the ear or 0.5–1.0 mg tid orally.
- Antihistamines: meclizine hydrochloride (Antivert), 25–100 mg per day in a divided dose, or dimenhydrinate (Dramamine), 50 mg qid
- Antiemetics: promethazine hydrochloride (Phenergan), 50–100 mg per day in a divided dose
- Benzodiazepines: diazepam or lorazepam
- Diuretics: hydrochlorothiazide, 50 mg per day

Caveat: All the above medications except diuretics have sedating effects and should be used only when necessary. Vestibular exercise, in which vertigo is induced by repeating the position to produce adaptation, is effective in treating mild vertigo (Brandt-Daroff exercise).

15

Primary Headaches and Facial Pain

EVALUATION OF THE PATIENT WITH HEADACHE

History

Obtaining a careful and thorough history is the most important part of the evaluation of a patient with headache. You should establish the following as you take the history:

- Age at onset of headache
- Onset of headache: acute, subacute, or chronic
- Severity and frequency of headache
- Characteristics of the pain as described by the patient
- Location and duration of headache
- Associated symptoms or signs
- Aggravating or relieving factors
- **Social history:** occupation, marital status, and history of alcohol or drug abuse

- **Family history:** this information is very important, because approximately 50% of patients with migraine have a positive family history
- **Medical history:** history of hypertension, depression, or glaucoma
- **Medication history:** oral contraceptives, weight loss pills, or medications that have been used to treat headache

Physical and Neurologic Examination

Examine the head and neck, record blood pressure, and check peripheral pulses. For any new patient, a complete neurologic examination is mandatory. Special attention is particularly given to the neck to check for stiffness, listening for bruits, fundoscopy examination, pupillary size and reactions, visual field, cranial nerves, and any focal neurologic signs.

Laboratory Tests

With a thorough history supplemented by careful examination, you can diagnose many headaches and facial pains with a high degree of certainty. In a few clinical conditions, discussed later in this chapter, laboratory tests are warranted.

TYPES OF HEADACHES

Tension-Type Headache

- Tension-type headache is the most common type of headache, affecting approximately 80% of patients presenting with headache. The onset is insidious, and pain increases as the day goes on. The pain is achy and dull and often starts from the occipital head region and spreads bifrontally or in a bandlike pattern. Tightness of the neck muscles is common.
- The headache may last from 30 minutes to several days and can occur daily or episodically.
- Some patients may give a history of migraine-type headaches in previous years.
- The pathophysiology is unknown, but stress or tension is a contributing factor.
- The neurologic examination is generally normal. In a typical case, there is no need for laboratory studies.
- **Treatment** includes daily exercise, muscle relaxation, and avoidance of alcohol and caffeine. Aspirin, acetaminophen, nonsteroidal anti-inflammatory drugs (NSAIDs), and tricyclic antidepressants (TCAs) are effective in the treatment of tension-type headache. Start TCAs in a low dose and build up to the adequate dose. Avoid polypharmacy, and do not use narcotic medication.

Migraine Headaches

Migraine with Aura

- Migraine with aura is common in middle-aged and educated women.
- Formerly called *classic migraine*, it causes a unilateral, intermittent, moderate to severe throbbing (pulsating, sharp) headache, particularly over the frontotemporal regions.
- A small percentage of patients complain of irritability, mood changes, or food cravings (e.g., chocolate) a few days before the headaches, which are considered premonitory symptoms.
- The onset of headache is usually acute; duration is between 4 and 72 hours.
- Migraine is commonly associated with nausea and vomiting, photophobia, and phonophobia; a patient with migraine headache prefers a dark, quiet room.
- The headache is aggravated by physical activity, menstruation, smoking, oral contraceptives, alcohol, cheese, monosodium glutamate, and processed foods.
- The aura manifests as visual symptoms such as hemianopia, flashing lights (photopsia), stars or spots, and, more characteristically, scintillating scotoma. Other less common auras include facial and arm paresthesia, speech difficulties, and weakness. Auras may occur singly or in combination and usually last 10–15 minutes.

- Migraine is now believed to be neuronal in origin, involving the brain stem, hypothalamus, and trigeminal system. An aura is due to neuronal suppression secondary to decreased cerebral blood flow originating from the occipital lobes, spreading anteriorly (spreading depression).

Migraine without Aura

Formerly called *common migraine*, migraine without aura is more common than migraine with aura. Its clinical presentation is the same but diffuse.

Complicated Migraine

- Complicated migraine is characterized by focal neurologic signs that persist 48–72 hours after the resolution of the headache.
- The most common forms of complicated migraine are ophthalmoplegic and hemiplegic migraine.
- Before the diagnosis of complicated migraine can be made, a structural lesion (e.g., arteriovenous malformation, aneurysm) should be excluded by a neuroimaging technique, unless the patient is known to you and has been previously investigated.

Migraine Infarction

Migraine infarction is a neurologic deficit that persists after the resolution of the headache. Stroke evaluation is required in these patients.

Basilar-Artery Migraine

Basilar-artery migraine is commonly seen in young girls manifesting as an occipital, throbbing headache associated with dizziness, blurred vision and diplopia, paresthesias, and even syncopal episodes. An electroencephalogram (EEG) should be obtained to rule out a seizure, and a magnetic resonance imaging (MRI) scan of the head should be obtained to rule out a posterior fossa or brain stem lesion.

Migraine Aura without Headache

Migraine aura without headache (acephalgic migraine) is characterized by the onset of a typical migraine aura (scintillating scotoma) but without the presence of a headache. In young adults this condition should be differentiated from a seizure by EEG. In the elderly, this condition should be differentiated from a transient ischemic attack through a stroke evaluation.

Treatment of Migraine

Nonpharmacologic

Nonpharmacologic treatment of migraine includes

- Avoidance of aggravating factors
- Biofeedback and relaxation techniques
- Regular daily exercise

It is important to establish a good relationship with the patient; migraineurs are generally sensitive and intelligent individuals. They want to know the cause of the headaches, the type of treatment, and the outcome. Set aside time for their questions in the evaluation.

Pharmacologic

NONSPECIFIC SYMPTOMATIC DRUG THERAPY
Nonspecific symptomatic treatment of migraine includes the use of

- NSAIDs
- Aspirin
- Acetaminophen
- Minor narcotics: hydrocodone or butorphanol (Stadol) in special cases
- Excedrin Migraine (over-the-counter)

ABORTIVE SYMPTOMATIC DRUG THERAPY
Abortive symptomatic treatment is given during an aura or before the peak of the headache on an as needed basis.

Ergotamines: Ergotamines may be given alone or in combination with caffeine (Cafergot, Ergostat). Ergotamines may be given orally or parenterally, as a suppository, or as a nasal spray. The maximum oral dose is 6 mg per day. Ergotamines are vasoconstrictors, and their antimigraine effects are mostly due to stimulation of the 5HT-1-D or 5HT-B receptors. These drugs are habit forming and can produce withdrawal headaches. Ergotamines are contraindicated in pregnancy and in patients with complicated migraine, hypertension, ischemic heart disease, and peptic ulcer disease. In the elderly patient, obtain an electrocardiogram before administering ergotamines.

Dihydroergotamine: Dihydroergotamine (DHE-45) is an agonist to 5HT-1-D and 5HT-1-B and other aminergics. This drug can be given intravenously (IV), intramuscularly, or subcutaneously (SC). It relieves the headache in 80% of patients and is a particularly good drug to use in severe or intractable migraine. The contraindications are the same as for ergotamines but the side effects are reduced, and it does not cause habituation. When administered IV, DHE-45 should be given with an antiemetic agent (metoclopramide [Reglan]). DHE-45 nasal spray (Migranal) is also available.

Serotonin Receptor Agonists: Serotonin receptor agonists include

- **Sumatriptan (Imitrex):** This is a specific 5HT-1-A and 5HT-1-B receptor agonist. It may be given orally, intra-muscularly or SC, and as a nasal spray. The maximum SC dose is 12 mg per day, and the maximum oral dose is 200 mg per day. Its side effects, contraindications, and precautions are the same as for the ergotamines.
- **Zolmitriptan (Zomig):** This enters the brain faster and stays longer than sumatriptan. The dose is 2.5 or 5.0 mg.

The starting dose is 2.5 mg, which is repeated in 2 hours. The dose should not exceed 10 mg within 24 hours.

- **Naratriptan (Amerge):** This drug, for prolonged and frequent attacks, is supplied as 1.0- and 2.5-mg tablets. The starting dose is 2.5 mg, followed by 1 mg every 4 hours, not to exceed 5 mg in a 24-hour period.
- **Rizatriptan (Maxalt):** The dosage is a 5- or 10-mg tablet and dissolving wafer. The 5-mg dose can be repeated if necessary every 2 hours, not to exceed 30 mg in a 24-hour period.
- **Isometheptene (Midrin):** Midrin is a combination of isometheptene plus dichloralphenazone and acetaminophen. The maximum dose is six capsules per day or 10 capsules per week. It has a bad taste and may elevate blood pressure.

PROPHYLACTIC DRUG THERAPY
Preventive therapy in migraine is indicated when headaches

- Are frequent (more than three per month)
- Are severe and disabling (i.e., interfere with work or household duties)
- Have no warning
- Are not responding to abortive or symptomatic treatment

Start prophylactic drugs with a low dose and titrate according to the patient's tolerance and response. These drugs should be given on a daily basis until an adequate response is achieved. Maintain at the lowest effective dose; the drugs may be discontinued after an adequate headache-free period. Be sure to know their side effects and contraindications. These drugs include

1. **Beta blockers**
   - Propranolol (Inderal), 20–360 mg per day
   - Atenolol, 25–150 mg per day
2. **TCAs**
   - Amitriptyline, 25–150 mg per day
   - Doxepin, 25–300 mg per day
3. **Antihistamines:** Cyproheptadine (Periactin), 4–40 mg per day
4. **Calcium channel blockers:** Verapamil, 80–400 mg per day
5. **NSAIDs:** Naproxen, 500–1,000 mg per day
6. **Antiserotonin drugs:** Methysergide (Sansert), 2–8 mg per day
7. **Antiepileptic drugs:** Divalproex (Depakote), 500–2,000 mg per day

Caveat: If the patient with suspected migraine does not respond to abortive treatment, consider other types of headaches or an underlying structural lesion.

Status Migrainosus

Status migrainosus results when repeated migraine headaches cause dehydration (due to nausea and vomiting). Most patients require brief hospitalization for treatment, which includes the following:

- Discontinuation of analgesics, sedatives, and narcotics
- Rehydration with IV fluids
- DHE-45, 0.5–1.0 mg IV, plus metoclopramide (Reglan), 10 mg IV q8h
- If the headaches persist, dexamethasone (4–10 mg qid IV) with benzodiazepine or ketorolac (30–60 mg) IV as needed

The **recommended protocol for repeated administration of DHE-45** is as follows:

- Premedicate with metoclopramide, 10 mg IV over 30 minutes.
- DHE-45, 0.5 mg IV over 1 minute.
- If headache improves, give DHE-45, 0.5 mg IV q8h as necessary.
- If headache improves but the patient has severe nausea, give metoclopramide or a lower dose of DHE-45 (0.15 mg).
- If headache persists and there is no nausea, give DHE-45, 0.5 mg IV q8h.

Cluster Headache

- Cluster headache is characterized by sudden onset of severe, intermittent, unilateral retro-orbital sharp pain.

- The pain is frequently associated with lacrimation and rhinorrhea on the same side as the pain.
- The headache lasts between 30 minutes and 3 hours and occurs as a cluster (i.e., several days to weeks with an interval of no headache).
- Partial Horner's syndrome is sometimes seen on the same side as the pain after the headache.
- During the pain, the patient prefers walking and pacing.
- The headache is precipitated by certain drugs (e.g., nitroglycerin) and alcohol and smoking.
- **Nonspecific symptomatic treatment** of cluster headache is the same as that for migraine.
- **Specific abortive treatment** includes
  - Oxygen (100% by mask) for 10–15 minutes
  - Sumatriptan (same as for migraine—see above)
  - Nasal lidocaine drops (4%)
  - Nasal sumatriptan
- **Prophylactic treatment** includes
  - Calcium channel blockers (verapamil)
  - Corticosteroids (60 mg per day for 3 days)
  - Lithium carbonate (300 mg tid) to provide a level of 0.7–1.2 mEq/liter (for chronic cluster headache)
  - Glycerol injection or gamma knife lesion of the trigeminal ganglion (for intractable cluster headache)

COMMON HEADACHE SYNDROMES

Chronic Daily Headache

Transformed Migraine

Transformed migraine is a chronic, frequent, migraine-like headache that does not respond to conventional anti-migraine drugs. Patients with transformed migraine often have mixed headaches (tension and migraine). Transformed migraine is probably the most common reason for a headache patient to seek a specialist.

Analgesic-Rebound Headache

Analgesic-rebound headache is another form of mixed headache and may occur when the patient overuses analgesics or medications that have butalbital (Fiorinal), benzodiazepines, or NSAIDs. Overnight, the patient develops withdrawal symptoms manifesting as headache in the morning. These patients should be detoxified before they respond to symptomatic or prophylactic medications.

Migraine during Pregnancy

Women with the onset of migraine during their menses or menarche usually improve when they become pregnant. Only a small percentage of these patients experience worsening headache. A new onset of migraine-like headache during the postpartum warrants further diagnostic evaluation to rule out sinus venous thrombosis, pseudotumor cerebri, and stroke.

Treatment of patients with migraine during pregnancy includes the following:

- Consulting a gynecologist
- Trying nonpharmacologic remedies
- Specific abortive treatments (Ergotamines, serotonin agonists, and Midrin should be avoided.)
- Nonspecific symptomatic treatments (Acetaminophen, NSAIDs, and minor narcotics may be used for a more severe headache.)
- Prophylactics (Propranolol and amitriptyline are to be used in lower doses if deemed necessary.)

Post-Traumatic Headache

Post-traumatic headaches are similar to tension or mixed-quality headaches. The pain is often diffuse or bifrontal and occurs after minor head trauma (concussion). These headaches are often associated with other symptoms of postconcussion syndrome (e.g., dizziness, fatigue, poor concentration). In uncomplicated cases (i.e., when there is no litigation), the headaches often resolve spontaneously in a few months.

Treatment of post-traumatic headaches includes nonspecific symptomatic therapy with aspirin, acetaminophen, NSAIDs, amitriptyline, or propranolol. Assurance is also important.

Pseudotumor Cerebri

- Pseudotumor cerebri causes a chronic, diffuse, dull, achy headache that is worse in the morning.
- Associated symptoms include visual obscuration and occasionally tinnitus and diplopia.
- The majority of patients are young, female, and overweight (with a recent change in weight).
- In uncomplicated cases, the neurologic examination is normal, except with the presence of bilateral papilledema.
- The pathophysiology of pseudotumor cerebri is not clearly understood but is thought to involve poor absorption of cerebrospinal fluid.
- In the **diagnostic evaluation**, computed tomography (CT) scan or MRI should be performed to rule out a space-occupying lesion or sinus venous thrombosis. Perform lumbar puncture (LP) to establish the high opening pressure (>28 mm Hg) and normal cerebrospinal composition.
- **Treatment** of pseudotumor cerebri includes the following:
  - Weight reduction (This change is effective but impractical most of the time.)
  - Nonspecific symptomatic (NSAIDs, acetaminophen, or TCAs).
  - Specific symptomatic (acetazolamide [Diamox], 250 mg qid; furosemide, 80 mg per day; or prednisone, 40 mg per day for several weeks).

- Repeat LP to reduce the opening pressure.
- Lumboperitoneal shunt and optic nerve sheath fenestration (decompression) when visual acuity decreases or the patient develops visual field defects.

Caveat: Patients with pseudotumor cerebri should be followed closely by a neurologist and an ophthalmologist. The goal of therapy is to not only control the headache but, more important, to save optic nerve function.

HOSPITALIZATION

Headaches that may require short-term hospitalization include

- First or worst headache of the patient's life
- Headache with a progressive course
- Headache associated with unexplained fever
- Headache associated with focal neurologic symptoms and signs other than typical aura
- Headache associated with the onset of seizures or prolonged mental confusion
- Status migrainosus, in which dehydration and pain need to be corrected with IV therapy

SPECIFIC DIAGNOSTIC TESTS

Headaches requiring specific diagnostic tests include

- **Pseudotumor cerebri:** MRI or CT scan of the brain, LP, complete blood cell count (CBC), erythrocyte sedimentation rate (ESR), thyroid-stimulating hormone level, thyroxine level

- **Temporal arteritis:** CBC, chemistry profile, ESR, temporal artery biopsy
- **Basilar-artery migraine:** EEG, MRI of the brain (to rule out a posterior fossa lesion)
- **Migraine with infarction, migraine with atypical or prolonged aura, or migraine that is unresponsive:** CBC; chemistry profile; ESR; MRI, magnetic resonance angiogram (MRA), or angiogram (when unruptured aneurysm, arteriovenous malformation, or vasculitis is suspected), carotid Doppler ultrasound, echocardiogram. In pregnant women with new-onset migraine or women who are postpartum, additional testing such as antiphospholipid antibody and protein C and S may be warranted (to rule out coagulopathy).
- **"First or worst headache of the life":** With this type of headache, particularly if associated with neck stiffness, nausea, vomiting, altered mental status, or focal neurologic signs, subarachnoid hemorrhage due to ruptured aneurysm should always be considered. Obtain a CT scan of the head; if negative, perform an LP. If the LP is negative in highly suspected cases, consider a four-vessel angiogram and neurosurgery consultation.
- **"Thunderclap headache":** A severe headache that reaches the maximum within a minute or so. Consider the possibility of an unruptured aneurysm and obtain at least an MRA. The same strategy is recommended for coital headaches.

- **Acute meningitis:** Neuroimaging followed by an LP.
- **Spontaneous internal carotid artery dissection:** Severe, unilateral periorbital headache, carotid bruits, Horner's syndrome, or focal neurologic symptoms and signs. Perform an MRI, MRA, or angiogram.

OPHTHALMOLOGY AND HEADACHES

Several headache syndromes are often associated with eye symptoms and signs:

- **Local eye disorder:** glaucoma, uveitis, cataract; considered as a cause of headaches in the elderly
- **Migraine headache:** photophobia, visual auras, ophthalmoplegia
- **Cluster headache:** ipsilateral (to pain) lacrimation, ipsilateral Horner's syndrome, photophobia
- **Pseudotumor cerebri:** visual obscuration, diplopia, blurred vision, photophobia, papilledema, visual field defect, decreased acuity (in untreated severe cases)
- **Temporal arteritis:** decreased visual acuity, visual field defect, ischemic optic neuritis
- **Subarachnoid hemorrhage:** photophobia, diplopia, papilledema, subhyaloid hemorrhage (pathognomonic if present)
- **Meningitis–focal encephalitis:** photophobia, papilledema, visual field defect
- **Cavernous sinus thrombosis:** ophthalmoplegia, proptosis, eye swelling

- **Tolosa-Hunt syndrome:** ophthalmoplegia (cavernous sinus granuloma)

FACIAL PAIN

Facial pain syndrome is caused by any pathologic condition arising from the face and mouth, such as sinusitis, dental infections, gum disease, throat infection, and temporomandibular joint dysfunction (syndrome). When the description of facial pain does not correlate with any known condition, either by history or examination, the term *atypical facial pain* is applied.

Trigeminal Neuralgia

- Trigeminal neuralgia (tic douloureux) is characterized by severe, sudden, paroxysmal, lancinating, unilateral facial pain of short duration (30–60 seconds) in the distribution of one or two branches of the trigeminal nerve (commonly V2 and V3).
- The pain is often triggered by touch, talking, swallowing, or brushing teeth. Immediately after the pain, transient facial numbness may occur.
- Trigeminal neuralgia is more common in middle-aged and elderly women. The pain is sometimes so severe it may induce facial grimacing (causing a tic).
- In younger individuals, the onset of trigeminal neuralgia may be seen with the onset of multiple sclerosis.

- The onset of trigeminal neuralgia in the young and a persistent motor or sensory deficit after pain warrants an MRI to exclude a brain stem lesion or multiple sclerosis.

Treatment

Medical
The drug of choice is carbamazepine (Tegretol), starting with a lower dose and titrating according to the response, aiming for a level of 8–11 mg per deciliter (600–1,200 mg/day). Other effective medications include

- Phenytoin, 300–400 mg per day
- Baclofen, 20–80 mg per day
- Clonazepam, 1–2 mg per day
- Amitriptyline, 50–100 mg per day
- Divalproex (Depakote), 1,000–1,500 mg per day
- Gabapentin (Neurontin), 2,400–3,600 mg per day

Surgical
Before considering surgical options, you may want to treat the patient with combination medication (polypharmacy). The surgical procedures include **gangliolysis** by radiofrequency or by infiltration of alcohol or glycerol. In selected cases repositioning of the compressing artery to the trigeminal nerve through a posterior fossa craniotomy may be considered (Jannetta procedure).

16

Peripheral Neuropathy

GENERAL CONSIDERATIONS

Peripheral neuropathy (PN) is a term applied to any condition affecting peripheral nerve function. When the disorder affects the peripheral nerve soma (motor or sensory neurons), the condition is known as a **neuronopathy**; when peripheral nerve fibers are affected, it is known as a neuropathy. Most peripheral nerves are mixed, having sensory motor and autonomic nerves. The pure form of sensory or motor neuropathy occurs when the soma (dorsal root ganglion or anterior horn cells) are selectively involved.

When evaluating a patient with suspected PN, a systematic approach is the best way to reach the diagnosis. Evaluation begins with careful history taking (history of neuropathy, past medical history, social history, family history, history of drugs, medication or toxic exposure, and occupational history). Physical examination begins with an evaluation of possible systemic illness, the skin, and any deformities of the bones or spine. Neurologic examination must be complete, with special attention to motor and sensory function. When approaching these patients, you should ask yourself

- **Does peripheral neuropathy exist?**
- **What is the cause of the neuropathy?**
- **What treatment can be offered to the patient?**

This chapter focuses on how to answer these questions. More comprehensive textbooks should be consulted for more detail on any particular neuropathies.

DOES A PERIPHERAL NEUROPATHY EXIST?

Not all patients complaining of "pins and needles," numbness, weakness, atrophy, or reflex changes have PN; therefore, it is important to establish the existence of PN first.

Clinical Features of Peripheral Neuropathy

Symptoms

Sensory
The most common symptoms of PN include pins and needles, or paresthesia, numbness, hypesthesia, dysesthesia, or unpleasant sensations; pain and burning; and decreased sensitivity to cold and warm. These symptoms typically begin in the distal lower extremities (toes) and gradually progress to the upper extremities and proximally. At the onset they may be asymmetric, focal, or symmetric. They may be intermittent or slowly progres-

sive. Some patients may even present with imbalance (sensory ataxia due to proprioception involvement).

Motor
Motor symptoms include complaints of weakness, muscle cramps, and fasciculation. Again, these symptoms usually begin in the distal lower extremities and progress proximally to the upper extremities. The extensor muscles are more affected than the flexors. Some neuropathies may begin proximally or start from the upper extremities. The onset may be symmetric or asymmetric. Patients typically complain of difficulty with dexterity and fine movement of the hands (e.g., turning a key, unbuttoning a shirt).

Autonomic
Autonomic symptoms include dizziness, dry eyes or mouth, an abnormal sweat pattern, persistent diarrhea, vomiting, and impotence.

Signs

Signs include decreased or absent sensory modalities (pain, touch, vibration, joint position) and Romberg's sign. The typical sensory deficits in a chronic generalized neuropathy have a "stocking-glove" distribution. The sensory deficit, however, could be in the distribution of one nerve (mononeuropathy) or multiple nerves (polyneuropathy or mononeuropathy multiplex). Preservation of proprioception suggests a small-fiber neuropathy (small myelinated or unmyelinated fibers). Some neuropathies may not present with a sensory deficit (e.g., motor neuropathies).

Motor
Motor signs include muscle weakness (distal more than proximal; extensors more than flexors), muscle atrophy (later stage), decreased or absent reflexes, normal or decreased muscle tone, fasciculation, and occasionally tremor (postural).

Autonomic
Autonomic signs include orthostatic hypotension; absence of heart rate variability in response to standing and deep breathing; sluggish pupillary reactions to light; Horner's syndrome; and dry mouth or eyes.

Other Important Signs
Any patient who presents with a neuropathy should be examined for skin and bone deformities or other systemic manifestations (e.g., systemic lupus erythematosus, sarcoidosis, thyroid problems). The following manifestations have particular diagnostic importance:

- **Palpable, hypertrophic nerve** (e.g., greater auricular, superficial peroneal): associated with hereditary neuropathies, chronic demyelinating neuropathies, amyloid neuropathy, and leprosy.
- **Skin lesions:** associated with porphyria, sarcoidosis, systemic lupus erythematosus, Fabry's disease, Refsum's disease, osteosclerotic myeloma (syndrome of

polyneuropathy, organomegaly, endocrinopathy, M protein, skin lesions [POEMS]), and arsenic poisoning.

- **Nail beds:** Mees' line is associated with arsenic and thallium poisoning; white nails are associated with POEMS.
- **Musculoskeletal:** Pes cavus and kyphoscoliosis are associated with hereditary neuropathies; hypertrophic muscle is associated with hereditary neuropathy and amyloidosis.

Electrophysiologic Diagnosis

Any patient with suspected PN should have electrophysiologic testing, which includes nerve conduction studies (NCSs) and needle electromyography (EMG). These tests help establish the existence of PN and also exclude other neuromuscular diseases affecting the motor unit. These tests can also indicate the pathology of PN, the distribution of PN, and the severity and evaluation of PN. Normal NCSs, however, do not rule out the presence of PN (e.g., small-fiber neuropathy or early stage of PN).

WHAT ARE THE CAUSES OF PERIPHERAL NEUROPATHY?

There are well over 100 causes of PN. Finding the cause of neuropathy can be the most difficult task for the practitioner. For practical purposes, there are two ways to find the cause.

Mnemonic Approach

The mnemonic DANG THERAPIST may be used to determine the cause of a PN:

D = diabetes

A = alcohol

N = nutritional deficiency (vitamin B_{12})

G = Guillain-Barré syndrome (GBS; the most common form of acute neuropathy in Western countries)

T = toxic (heavy metals or drugs) or metabolic (thyroid, liver, kidney disease)

H = hereditary (hereditary motor sensory neuropathies [HMSNs])

E = environmental

R = recurrent (acute intermittent porphyria [AIP], chronic inflammatory demyelinating polyneuropathy [CIDP])

A = amyloid

P = porphyria

I = inflammatory (GBS, CIDP, Lyme disease, human immunodeficiency virus [HIV], vasculitis, paraproteinemia)

S = systemic diseases

T = tumor (paraneoplastic neuropathy, a remote effect of carcinoma)

The most common types of HMSNs are

• HMSN I: Charcot-Marie-Tooth (CMT), demyelinating form

- HMSN II: CMT, neuronal (axonal) form
- HMSN III: Dejerine-Sottas disease
- HMSN IV: Refsum's disease
- HMSN V: Friedreich's ataxia

Classification Approach

PNs are classified in many ways. The following classification is probably the most useful and easy to memorize for the purposes of identifying the cause and planning a logical evaluation.

I. *Acute Neuropathies*

Acute Mononeuropathies
The acute mononeuropathies include the following:

- **Acute peroneal nerve palsy** commonly presents with footdrop, and on examination, there is weakness of foot dorsiflexors and evertors, with or without sensory deficit. Reflexes are usually preserved. Peroneal palsy must be differentiated from L5 radiculopathy or sciatic neuropathy. An underlying generalized neuropathy should also be excluded.
- **Acute radial nerve palsy** presents with wristdrop without significant sensory deficit. The site of the lesion is either at the spinal groove of the humerus or at the forearm (dorsal interosseus nerve). In children, wristdrop raises the possibility of lead intoxication; in adults, it is usually seen in alcoholics.

- **Acute seventh nerve (Bell's) palsy** is a common clinical entity. Decreased tearing and taste and hypersensitivity to sound (hyperacusis) usually implies proximal nerve involvement and an unfavorable prognosis. Protect the cornea from dryness and ulceration. Corticosteroids may expedite the recovery if administered within the first week.
- **Acute third nerve palsy** presents with acute eye pain on movement, ptosis, and diplopia. Pupillary responses are typically preserved. The common causes are diabetes and atherosclerosis.

Acute Polyneuropathies
Acute polyneuropathies include the following:

- Acute inflammatory demyelinating polyneuropathy or GBS (see Chapter 29)
- Acute toxic or metabolic neuropathies
- Acute intermittent porphyria
- Infectious neuropathies: Lyme disease, HIV, diphtheria

II. *Subacute, Chronic, Symmetric Sensorimotor Polyneuropathies*

The category of subacute neuropathies includes the most common forms and imposes diagnostic challenges to the clinician. It includes polyneuropathies associated with diabetes, alcohol use, nutritional deficiency (vitamin B_{12}), and paraproteinemias. It also includes amyloid, toxin- or

drug-induced, paraneoplastic, and multifocal motor neuropathies (MMNs).

III. *Mononeuropathy Multiplex*

The neuropathies in the mononeuropathy multiplex category present with involvement of different single nerves
at different sites and at different times. The best example
is the presentation of wristdrop followed by footdrop
and, later, a median neuropathy. The causes include diabetes, vasculitis, leprosy, HIV, and sarcoidosis.

IV. *Relapsing and Remitting Neuropathies*

Relapsing and remitting neuropathies include CIDP, AIP,
and MMNs.

V. *Hereditary Polyneuropathies*

Hereditary polyneuropathies include HMSN types I–V,
hereditary neuropathy with pressure palsy (HNPP), and
hereditary neuropathies due to enzyme deficiencies or
metabolic disorders.

VI. *Entrapment Neuropathies*

Common entrapment neuropathies include the following:

- **Carpal tunnel syndrome:** median nerve compression at
  the wrist
- **Cubital tunnel syndrome:** ulnar nerve compression at
  the elbow

- **Tarsal tunnel syndrome:** tibialis nerve entrapment in the tarsal tunnel of the foot
- **Meralgia paresthetica:** entrapment of the lateral femoral cutaneous nerve beneath the inguinal ligament or in the pelvis; presents with patchy paresthesias of the lateral aspect of the thigh

NEUROPATHY EVALUATION

Evaluation of suspected PN includes the following:

1. *Nerve conduction studies and needle EMG.* These tests should be done in all patients suspected of having neuropathies, not only to establish the existence of neuropathy but also to help you plan further evaluation.
2. *Routine or nonspecific evaluations.* The following studies are done in all patients with neuropathies: complete blood cell count, erythrocyte sedimentation rate, chemistry profile, serum protein electrophoresis and immune fixation, and vitamin B_{12} level (serum methylmalonic acid and homocysteine level are more specific than vitamin B_{12} level, but they cost more).
3. *Selective evaluations.* More selective evaluation is based on the NCS/EMG results and classification:
   a. **Acute mononeuropathies:** routine evaluation
   b. **Acute generalized polyneuropathies**
      (1) GBS: NCS plus lumbar puncture (to show elevated protein without increase in cells)

    (2)   Heavy metal intoxication: urine and serum lead levels and mercury levels

    (3)   Porphyria: Porphobilinogen deaminase level of red blood cells

    (4)   HIV: cerebrospinal fluid (CSF) analysis, HIV antibody, CD4 count

    (5)   Lyme disease: CSF analysis, Lyme disease antibodies

c. **Chronic, symmetric polyneuropathy:** routine evaluations and a few selected studies in some cases; anti-Hu antibody; chest computed tomographic scan for paraneoplastic neuropathy in men; protein electrophoresis; abdominal fat or nerve biopsy in case of amyloidosis

d. **Mononeuropathy multiplex:** erythrocyte sedimentation rate, rheumatoid factor, antinuclear antibody, C-reactive protein, cryoglobulins, angiotensin-converting enzyme level, chest x-ray, hemoglobin A_{1C}, muscle and nerve biopsy (superficial peroneal and peroneus brevis muscle), skin and nerve biopsy (leprosy)

e. **Relapsing and remitting neuropathies:** same evaluations as for acute generalized neuropathies

f. **Hereditary neuropathies:** DNA analysis (CMT1A) for CMT and HNPP; sural nerve biopsy in selected cases; lumbar puncture, plasma phytanic acid level, and nerve biopsy in suspected Refsum's disease (increased serum phytanic level)

g. **Entrapment neuropathies:** Complete blood cell count, chemistry, erythrocyte sedimentation rate, thyroid function tests (thyroid-stimulating hormone and thyroxine)

WHAT TREATMENT CAN BE OFFERED TO THE PATIENT?

Specific Therapy

Specific therapy includes the following:

- Vasculitic neuropathies, CIDP, MMN, and paraprotein neuropathies: prednisone and immunosuppressive drugs
- GBS, CIDP, and paraprotein neuropathies: plasma exchange, intravenous immune globulin
- Leprosy, Lyme disease, and HIV: antimicrobials and antiretrovirus drugs
- Refsum's disease: low phytanic acid diet
- Correcting underlying metabolic or systemic disease (diabetes, thyroid, kidney, etc.)
- Heavy metal neuropathies: chelating therapy, penicillamine
- AIP: high-carbohydrate diet with 3 mg/kg/day of hematin (Panhematin) for 4 days during an attack

- Vitamin B_{12} deficiency: 100 µg of B_{12} intramuscularly twice weekly for 4 weeks, then weekly for 3 months and monthly thereafter

Symptomatic Therapy

Symptomatic therapy for the pain and paresthesia of PN includes the following:

- For sharp, lancinating pain (**epicritic pain**): carbamazepine (Tegretol); baclofen; prazosin; gabapentin; mexiletine, 200 mg per day for 3 days, increase to 200–400 mg tid (assess the heart first)
- For burning, deep pain (**protopathic pain**): amitriptyline; desipramine (Norpramin); nortriptyline (Pamelor); capsaicin (Zostrix) ointment, 3–4 times per day (may be mixed with 5% EMLA cream)

PN patients may also receive occupational and physical therapy. Surgery may be performed on patients with entrapment and compressive neuropathies.

CLINICAL CLUES TO SOME NEUROPATHIES

- CMT: pes cavus, hammer toes, reverse "champagne bottle appearance" of legs ("stork legs")
- Refsum's disease: scaly, dry skin (ichthyosis); retinitis pigmentosa; hearing loss; cataract; cardiac conduction defect

- Fabry's disease: angiokeratoma (reddish maculopapular rash in the umbilical and groin areas), kidney failure
- Arsenic poisoning: hyperkeratosis, pink hands, scaly skin of the soles and palms, Mees' line on the fingernail beds
- POEMS syndrome: peripheral neuropathy (P), white nails, clubbing, organomegaly (O), endocrinopathy (E) (gynecomastia, testicular atrophy), M protein (M), hyperpigmentation of the skin (S)

17

Movement Disorders

Movement disorders typically result from abnormalities of the extrapyramidal system. The core structures of the extrapyramidal system include the caudate nucleus, globus pallidus, substantia nigra, red nucleus, and subthalamic nucleus and their connections to the frontal cortex, brain stem, and cerebellum. This chapter describes the approach to common movement disorders.

EVALUATION

In history taking, you should determine the patient's age at onset, the family history, and any history of neuropsychiatric illness or neuroleptic drug use. In the neurologic examination, pay attention to the type of movement disorder and any associated neurologic findings.

DIAGNOSIS: TERMINOLOGY OF ABNORMAL MOVEMENTS

The most important aspect of evaluating a movement disorder is recognizing the general category of abnormal movements and then planning your additional diagnostic testing. It is important to learn the following terminology used to describe abnormal movements:

- **Tremor:** rhythmic involuntary oscillation of a body part. Usually involves the distal extremities and often starts in the dominant hand. Tremor is subclassified according to the position of the limb (rest, action, intention, postural).
- **Chorea:** rapid, irregular, brief, purposeless movements, often involving a distal limb.
- **Athetosis:** slow, irregular, undulating, writhing-type movement, often associated with chorea.
- **Tics:** stereotyped, irregular, simple, or complex forceful movements.
- **Dystonia:** sustained, abnormal contraction of a group of muscles resulting in abnormal posture of the limb.
- **Ballismus:** violent, flinging movements, often involving a proximal limb, usually unilateral (hemiballismus), due to a contralateral subthalamic nucleus lesion.
- **Myoclonus:** sudden, irregular shock-like contraction of the muscle or group of muscles.
- **Tardive dyskinesia:** stereotyped movements often involving the facial and oral muscles, manifesting as tongue protrusion, chewing, lip smacking, and facial grimacing. This condition is seen after chronic use of dopamine blockers neuroleptics.
- **Rigidity:** increased muscle tone throughout the passive range of motion of the limb. When there is coexistence

of tremor, the examiner detects a ratchety resistance, referred to as "cogwheel rigidity."

PARKINSON'S DISEASE

Parkinson's disease (PD) is the most common movement disorder and is caused by slowly progressive degeneration of the dopaminergic neurons of the substantia nigra. Dopamine depletion accounts for most symptoms of PD. The prevalence of PD is approximately 1–2% of people older than age 70. The average age of onset is 55 years, but patients in their 20s are also reported.

Clinical Features

The cardinal features of PD include

- **Resting tremor:** 4- to 7-Hz, coarse, pill-rolling tremor. The tremor usually starts unilaterally (in the dominant hand) and sometimes involves the legs. The tremor diminishes with action and is exacerbated at rest, during physical and mental activities, and while walking.
- **Cogwheel rigidity:** Usually presents in the affected limb and neck. The rigidity is increased by contralateral repeated movements (e.g., finger tapping).
- **Bradykinesia:** slowness of voluntary movements such as diminished arm swing during walking, masked face, diminished blinking and micrographia. Limb bradykinesia is seen during finger tapping. The amplitude and

speed of the movements will decrease the longer the movement is performed.

- **Postural instability:** stooped posture, short-stepped walking, shuffling, festination, and frequent falls. The motor signs of PD are usually asymmetric and responsive to levodopa.
- **Other symptoms and signs:** depression, personality changes, psychosis and dementia, sialorrhea, facial seborrhea, autonomic dysfunction, dysphagia, and constipation.

Differential Diagnosis

The differential diagnosis of PD includes

- Essential tremor
- Drug-induced parkinsonism
- Parkinsonism due to environmental toxins
- Other degenerative conditions: progressive supranuclear palsy, multiple system atrophy (which includes striatonigral degeneration, Shy-Drager syndrome, and olivopontocerebellar degeneration), cortical-basal ganglionic degeneration, normal pressure hydrocephalus, and Wilson's disease

Management

The management of PD is complex. Early and mild PD can be treated by general practitioners, but more advanced stages of the disease are best handled by a neurologist with a special interest and expertise in PD. I provide general guidelines below, but you should refer to neurology textbooks for more detail.

What You Should Know

- The goal of therapy is to improve the patient's quality of life and disability as much as possible with the lowest effective dose of medication.
- Treatment of PD is threefold: pharmacologic, surgical, and nonpharmacologic.
- PD is a chronic, progressive disease.
- After choosing a medication for a patient, "start low, go slow."
- Age is the most important factor in determining when and how to initiate therapy.
- Because polypharmacy is often needed in patients with PD, change one drug at a time.
- Misdiagnosis of PD is common and treatment is complex, so patients suspected of having PD are best evaluated and treated by a movement disorder specialist.
- Patients with PD often have other problems that should be addressed and treated, such as constipation, urinary problems, sexual problems, orthostatic hypotension, dementia, psychosis, hallucinations, and a variety of sleep disorders.

Pharmacotherapy

- Pharmacotherapy should be tailored individually according to the patient's symptoms and their severity, the patient's age, and whether cognitive function is impaired.
- Levodopa is the most effective drug to treat all manifestations of PD, but its use should be delayed as long as possible in patients younger than 70 years to impede its adverse motor side effects (fluctuations and dyskinesias).
- Rational polypharmacy is justified in more severe cases.
- You should be familiar with the drugs that are used in PD and their dosages, side effects, and indications.
- The following drugs are commonly used in the United States:
  - **Anticholinergics:** benztropine mesylate (Cogentin; 0.5–1.0 mg per day, up to 8 mg per day), trihexyphenidyl mesylate (Artane; 1 mg at bedtime, up to 6 mg per day in divided doses)
  - **Dopaminergic and anticholinergic:** amantadine hydrochloride (Symmetrel; 100 mg bid or tid)
  - **Monoamine oxidase B inhibitor:** selegiline (Deprenyl, Eldepryl; 5 mg bid)
  - **Levodopa/carbidopa** (Sinemet and controlled-release Sinemet)
  - **Dopamine agonists**
    - Ergot derived

- Bromocriptine (Parlodel; 2.5 mg [one-half tablet] bid, up to 30–40 mg per day)
- Pergolide (Permax; 0.05 mg × 2 days, max dose is 3–5 mg per day)
- Nonergot derived
  - Pramipexole (Mirapex; 0.125 mg tid, increase gradually, max dose is 4.5 mg per day in three divided doses)
  - Ropinirole (Requip; 0.25 mg tid, max dose is 8 mg tid)
- **Catechol methyltransferase inhibitors:** tolcapone (Tasmar), 100–200 mg tid

Surgery

Medial pallidotomy by stereotactic technique may be considered for patients in the advanced stage of the disease and significant disability despite medical therapy. Other surgical procedures include thalamotomy, deep-brain stimulation, and fetal-cell transplants.

ESSENTIAL TREMOR

Clinical Features

- Essential tremor (ET) is usually a bilateral but asymmetric tremor affecting the hands, neck, head, and jaw and sometimes the tongue.
- Tremor of the neck and tongue may affect speech and swallowing.

- The tremor is worse when a limb is in action (e.g., writing, reading, drawing, drinking) and postural (e.g., outstretched arms).
- The term *benign essential tremor* may not be appropriate, because the tremor can be very disabling.
- There is usually strong family history in ET patients.
- The onset may occur when the patient is in middle age or after age 65.
- The tremor should exist for at least 5 years and other causes should be excluded before the diagnosis of ET can be made.
- Characteristically, some patients show favorable response to a small amount of alcohol.

Treatment

Pharmacotherapy

- Propranolol (Inderal) is the drug of choice; start the long-acting form at 60 mg per day and increase to 80 mg per day if necessary. Up to 320 mg of regular Inderal may be given.
- Primidone (Mysoline) may be used in patients who cannot take Inderal. However, most patients cannot tolerate the sedation side effects of primidone. Start with a very low dose (25 mg qhs) and increase when necessary.
- Use of alcohol (e.g., red wine) before a meal at social events may be considered in some patients. Addiction to this form of therapy is somewhat overstated.

- **Other medications for treating ET include**
  - Clonazepam (Klonopin)
  - Gabapentin (Neurontin)
  - Acetazolamide (Diamox)
  - Calcium channel blockers (verapamil)
  - Botulinum toxin injection (Botox)

Surgery

Stereotactic thalamotomy (unilateral) or thalamic stimulation (bilateral) may be considered for intractable disabling tremor.

DRUG-INDUCED EXTRAPYRAMIDAL SYNDROMES

Suspect drug-induced movement disorders in patients receiving antipsychotic medications, particularly dopamine blockers, and patients living in a psychiatric institution. Common drug-induced extrapyramidal syndromes include tremor, dystonia, akathisia, parkinsonism, and tardive dyskinesia.

Neuroleptics with a high incidence of producing extrapyramidal syndromes include

- Haloperidol (Haldol)
- Fluphenazine (Prolixin)
- Trifluoperazine (Stelazine)

Neuroleptics with the least incidence of producing extrapyramidal syndromes include

- Clozapine (Clozaril)
- Quetiapine (Seroquel)
- Olanzapine (Zyprexa)
- Thioridazine (Mellaril)
- Risperidone (Risperdal)

Other medications include

- Metoclopramide (Reglan)
- Prochlorperazine (Compazine)
- Promethazine (Phenergan)

Acute Drug-Induced Dystonia

Acute drug-induced dystonia features abnormal tongue posture and neck dystonia. It occurs within the first 3 days of starting a neuroleptic. Treatment includes benztropine (Cogentin), 2 mg intravenously or intramuscularly, or diphenhydramine (Benadryl), 50 mg intravenously.

Tardive Dyskinesia

Patients with tardive dyskinesia experience abnormal oral, buccal, or lingual movement after chronic use (i.e., ≥6 months) of dopamine blockers. **Treatment** includes gradual reduction of neuroleptics if possible and the following:

- Reserpine (Serpasil): This drug depletes central nervous system biogenic amines. Begin at 0.25 mg per day and increase to 2–4 mg per day if necessary.
- Divalproex (Depakote), 500–2,500 mg per day
- Clonazepam (Klonopin), 1–2 mg per day
- Baclofen, 10–30 mg per day
- Diazepam, 5–20 mg per day
- Vitamin E, 400–800 mg per day

MYOCLONUS

Most patients with myoclonus are treated with clonazepam and/or divalproex (Depakote).

18

Sleep Disorders

Recognition of sleep disorders is important because

- They are common, affecting approximately 10–15% of the U.S. population.
- Many medical, neurologic, and psychiatric disorders present with sleep problems.
- Sleep disorders can have a significant impact on a patient's physical, social, and occupational life.

SLEEP: THE BASICS

Nonrapid Eye Movement Sleep

The features of non–rapid eye movement (NREM) sleep include the following:

1. Electroencephalographic features:
   - Stage 1: drowsiness, disappearance of alpha wave, mild slowing of background
   - Stage 2: light sleep, spindle wave, vertex-sharp wave, K complexes
   - Stages 3 and 4: deep sleep, slow waves (theta and delta)

2. Decreased body temperature, increased vagal tone
3. Normal muscle tone
4. Increased growth hormone secretion

Rapid Eye Movement Sleep

The features of rapid eye movement (REM) sleep include the following:

1. Electroencephalographic features: similar to stage 1 NREM; presence of rapid, jerky eye movements; sawtooth waves
2. Decreased muscle tone except extraocular muscles, diaphragm, and occasional limb jerks
3. Increased autonomic activities: increased body temperature, increased basal metabolic rate, increased blood pressure, pupillary dilation, sweating, irregular breathing, increased brain activity and cerebral blood flow
4. Penile erection
5. Dreaming

Sleep Cycles

In adults, sleep begins with NREM. The first REM sleep occurs within 70–90 minutes, and successive REM sleep occurs every 90 minutes. Four to six REM cycles occur during 7–8 hours of night sleep. In adults, REM sleep constitutes approximately 20% of total sleep. After age 60 years, there are virtually no stages 3 and 4 of NREM sleep.

Biological Rhythms

Circadian rhythms cycle approximately every 24 hours, but in most of us, sleep-awake cycles are approximately 25 hours long (ultradian).

Neuroanatomy

Raphe nuclei in the pons are the source of NREM, and the nucleus gigantocellularis of the pons is the source of REM. Serotonin is a major neurotransmitter for sleep.

SPECIFIC SLEEP DISORDERS

Insomnias

Insomnia is defined as chronic lack of adequate sleep to maintain normal daytime function. Transient insomnia is common. Chronic insomnia can be caused by medical, neurologic, psychiatric, or drug or alcohol problems, or it may be idiopathic. Most parasomnias are associated with insomnia. Treatment depends on the underlying cause. Low doses of sedative-hypnotic medications (benzodiazepines) are used for disabling insomnias.

Excessive Daytime Sleepiness: Narcolepsy

The incidence of narcolepsy is 1:1,000 to 1:10,000. The age at onset is 20–40 years. Narcolepsy is strongly associated with HLA-DR15 and HLA-DQW6.

Clinical Features

The clinical features of narcolepsy include

- Excessive daytime sleepiness manifested as a sleep attack that lasts 10–15 minutes while the patient is sedentary. The patient is often refreshed on awakening.
- Cataplexy: sudden onset of hypotonia after an exciting event (e.g., laughter, anger) lasting a few minutes. Eye and respiratory muscles are usually spared.
- Sleep paralysis: generalized weakness during falling asleep or on awakening, lasting a few minutes; may be frightening.
- Hypnagogic hallucination: vivid (auditory or visual) hallucination during sleep or on waking. In narcolepsy, sleep begins with REM (sleep-onset REM), causing dysregulation in the sleep-awake cycle. Diagnosis is made by history, sleep studies, and HLA typing.

Treatment

Treatment of narcolepsy includes the following:

- Sleep attacks: methylphenidate (Ritalin), 5–60 mg per day; dextroamphetamine, 5–60 mg per day; or pemoline, up to 75–100 mg per day

- Cataplexy and sleep paralysis: tricyclic antidepressant (Tofranil, 50–200 mg/day), pemoline (up to 75 mg/day), or fluoxetine (20–80 mg per day)

Sleep Apnea Syndrome

Sleep apnea syndrome features cessation of breathing during sleep.

Clinical Features

Obstructive sleep apnea is seen in obese, middle-aged men with short necks, micrognathia, or enlarged tonsils or adenoids. In these patients thoracic movement is intact, but there is no air flow through the nose during sleep. The **symptoms** of obstructive sleep apnea are early morning headache, excessive daytime sleepiness, fatigue, poor concentration, and a loud snore or snort during sleep after an apneic event. Frequent and prolonged apnea is more serious.

Central sleep apnea syndrome features cessation of chest and upper air flow during sleep. Its symptoms are similar to those of obstructive sleep apnea. The cause is unknown.

Mixed sleep apnea syndrome is a combination of both syndromes.

Complications

The complications of sleep apnea syndrome include

- Cardiac arrhythmia

- Hypoxia
- Pulmonary hypertension
- Right heart failure
- Hypertension
- Stroke
- Polycythemia
- Asystole

Treatment

Treatment of sleep apnea syndrome includes

- Weight loss
- Diuretics: Diamox, up to 1,000 mg per day
- Antidepressants
- Aminophylline
- Continuous positive airway pressure or bilevel positive airway pressure
- Tracheotomy

PARASOMNIAS

Parasomnias often feature abnormal behavior occurring exclusively during sleep or exacerbated by sleep.

Nonrapid Eye Movement Sleep Parasomnias

Enuresis

Bedwetting beyond age 5 is abnormal. It occurs primarily during stage 3 and 4 NREM sleep. Primary cases are usually due to neurologic or maturational lag and often are hereditary. Secondary cases are due to urologic, psychological, or medical (e.g., diabetes) problems. **Treatment** is with low-dose imipramine, tricyclic antidepressants, or behavioral therapy.

Sleep Walking

Sleep walking, or somnambulism, is a complex behavior characterized by walking, climbing, and running during stages 3 and 4 of NREM sleep. When the patient is awakened, he or she is confused. The onset is in childhood and disappears after adolescence. Patients who sleep walk should be protected from self injury.

Sleep Talking

Sleep talking, or somniloquy, is a common problem. It may be associated with sleep walking.

Bruxism

Patients with bruxism grind their teeth at night.

Night Terrors

Night terrors, or pavor nocturnus, feature the sudden onset of a scream or cry. They are associated with autonomic hyperactivation: tachycardia, tachypnea, and sweating. If awakened, the patient is confused and has no recollection of the event. Night terrors are common in childhood and disappear by adolescence. They may lead to serious injury.

Sleep Myoclonus

Sleep myoclonus, or hypnic jerks, occur during stages 1 and 2 of NREM sleep. Treatment is low-dose clonazepam (0.5–1.0 mg) at bedtime.

Periodic Limb Movements

Periodic limb movements are stereotyped, rhythmic head or limb movements seen most frequently in children. Benzodiazepines or antidepressants may be given for treatment.

Post-Traumatic Stress Disorder

Patients with post-traumatic stress disorder have subjective sleep complaints, flashbacks, or nightmares. Any emotional trauma may lead to post-traumatic stress disorder.

Restless Legs Syndrome

Restless legs syndrome causes an unpleasant, indescribable sensation of the legs, resulting in an irresistible urge to move the limb. It is often associated with nocturnal myoclonus and has a strong familial occurrence. The drug of choice is clonazepam (0.5–1.0 mg/day) at night. Other drugs include temazepam (Restoril), carbamazepine, and carbidopa-levodopa (Sinemet).

Rapid Eye Movement Sleep Parasomnias

Rapid Eye Movement Sleep Disorder

REM behavior sleep disorder (RBD) is a recently described sleep disorder characterized by often violent behavior such as kicking, punching, yelling, and running during REM sleep. Patients with RBD appear to be acting on their dreams; in these individuals hypotonia or atonia during REM does not occur. RBD is suspected when the patient or his or her sleep partner complains of injury during sleep. The patient has no control or recollection of the behavior during sleep. RBD is commonly associated with degenerative diseases of the central nervous system such as Parkinson's disease, Huntington's disease, olivopontocerebellar atrophy, dementias, multisystem atrophy, and spinocerebellar degeneration. The drug of choice is clonazepam, with a starting dose of 0.5–1.0 mg at night. If the patient does not respond to clonazepam, imipramine, carbamazepine, clonidine, Sinemet, or gabapentin may be tried.

Nightmares

Nightmares are frightening dreams that usually awaken the patient from REM sleep. They occur at any age and may be associated with medical or psychological problems. Nightmares should be differentiated from complex partial seizures. Treatment involves behavioral therapy and correcting any underlying medical illness. The drug of choice is cyproheptadine (Periactin), 4–24 mg at night.

Sinus Cardiac Arrest

Sinus cardiac arrest during REM sleep has recently been described in the literature. These patients may present with early morning lightheadedness, blurred vision, or chest pain. The condition may be related to autonomic hyperactivity during REM. In the severe form, the patient may require a pacemaker.

Impaired or Painful Penile Erection

Impairment of penile erection or painful erection is a disorder occurring during REM sleep that primarily affects middle-aged men.

SLEEP-AWAKE (CIRCADIAN) SLEEP DISORDERS

Sleep-awake cycle disorders are caused by jet lag and shift work. Patients with delayed sleep phase syndrome go to sleep late and wake up early in the morning.

DIAGNOSIS OF SLEEP DISORDERS

To diagnose a sleep disorder, obtain a detailed history (medical, psychological, drug), perform a complete neurologic examination, and have the patient complete a detailed questionnaire and record a sleep diary log.

Sleep studies, such as a multiple sleep latency test and polysomnography, should be considered in chronic, primary sleep disorder, particularly in patients with cardiopulmonary dysfunction (sleep apnea), movement disorders, RBD, narcolepsy, or impairment of penile erection (impotence). Not all sleep disorders require polysomnography for diagnosis. See Chapter 7 for a description of the multiple sleep latency test and polysomnography.

19

Neuromuscular Diseases

ANATOMY: THE BASICS

The **motor unit** is the anatomic core of the peripheral nervous system. It consists of motor neurons or **anterior horn cells**, and **muscle fibers** that are inverted by their peripheral nerve axons. Peripheral nerve axons are either myelinated or unmyelinated. The majority of autonomic fibers are unmyelinated. Other parts of the motor unit are the nerve root, plexus, and neuromuscular junction. Knowing the components of the motor unit will help you locate the site of pathology in the peripheral nervous system.

The number of motor units in muscles differs according to the size of the muscles. In eye muscles, one anterior horn cell innervates approximately 10 muscle fibers, whereas in thigh muscles one anterior horn cell innervates as many as 2,000 fibers.

Muscle fibers consist of myofibrils, which have thousands of myofilaments. Myofilaments are contractile proteins (actin and myosin). Each muscle fiber has one neuromuscular junction structure (end-plate zone). You should know the structure and function of the neuromuscular junction.

In a histochemistry study, a muscle biopsy specimen, when stained with adenosine triphosphatase (preincubation pH = 9.4), will show two distinct muscle fiber types. Type 1 fibers stain light brown, and type 2 fibers stain dark brown. Type 1 fibers are red, aerobic, oxidative, and fatigue resistant. Type 2 fibers are white, anaerobic, glycolytic, and fatigable. The two types are equally distributed in a checkerboard pattern.

EVALUATION OF THE PATIENT WITH NEUROMUSCULAR DISEASE

The **history** is a very important part of the evaluation of a patient with neuromuscular disease. Do not forget family history and a list of prescribed medications.

Common Symptoms of Neuromuscular Disease

- Weakness and fatigue
- Sensory complaints
- Myalgia and cramps
- Falling and difficulty walking

Common Signs

- Weakness, which may be focal, unilateral, or diffuse; predominantly proximal or distal; symmetric or asymmetric; progressive or fluctuating

- Muscle bulk: normal, atrophy, or hypertrophy
- Sensory deficit: normal, decreased, or increased
- Muscle tone: normal, hypotonia, or hypertonia
- Reflex changes: normal, decreased, or increased
- Spontaneous movements: fasciculation (muscle twitches), myokymia (undulating muscle contractions), or cramps

Commonly Performed Diagnostic Tests for Patients with Neuromuscular Disease

- **Blood tests:** complete blood cell count (CBC), chemistry profile, serum creatine kinase (CK), erythrocyte sedimentation rate (ESR), thyroid function tests, serum autoantibodies, and DNA analysis. The blood tests chosen depend on the suspected cause.
- **Electrophysiologic tests:** Nerve conduction studies (NCSs), needle electromyography (EMG), repetitive nerve stimulation, and single-fiber EMG.
- **Imaging:** chest x-rays, chest computed tomography (CT), and other imaging techniques depending on the suspected cause.
- **Lumbar puncture** in selected cases.
- **Muscle or nerve biopsy** in selected cases.

DIAGNOSIS

The best way to reach a diagnosis or plan your evaluation is to try to localize the site of pathology along the **motor unit. Ask yourself**, "Is the disorder due to the anterior horn cell, a plexus lesion, peripheral neuropathy, neuromuscular junction disease, or muscle disease (myopathy)?"

Clinical Characteristics of Motor Neuron Disease

The clinical characteristics of motor neuron disease (e.g., amyotrophic lateral sclerosis [ALS]) include

- Weakness and muscle atrophy: more prominent in distal muscles and often asymmetric. The bulbar muscles are generally affected (manifesting as dysarthria or dysphagia); the ocular muscles are generally spared. The weakness is progressive ("creeping paralysis").
- Sensory complaints or deficit: usually absent or minimal.
- Muscle tone: generally increased.
- Generalized persistent fasciculation (do not forget to look at the tongue for atrophy and fasciculation).
- Reflexes: hyperactive, but may diminish when there is severe muscle wasting.
- Plantar responses: often extensor (Babinski's sign).
- Mental status; eye movements; and sensory, autonomic, bladder, and sexual function: generally normal.

Clinical Characteristics of Nontraumatic, Adult-Onset Brachial Plexitis

- Onset of severe shoulder pain (worse with movement)
- Weakness and sensory deficit: referable to the affected nerves

- Unilateral
- Depressed reflexes
- Muscle atrophy in later stage
- Upper trunk of plexus usually affected

Clinical Characteristics of Polyneuropathies

- Sensory symptoms and deficits, which usually begin at the distal limbs and may progress proximally
- Motor weakness and wasting: distal muscles are greatly involved
- Motor and sensory features, which may be symmetric or asymmetric in distribution
- Reflexes: often diminished or absent
- Muscle tone: either normal or decreased

Clinical Characteristics of Neuromuscular Junction Disorder (e.g., Myasthenia Gravis)

- Weakness and fatigue in the distribution of the oculo-bulbar or limb muscles
- Weakness fluctuates: improves with rest, worsens with use
- Muscle tone, sensory examination, and reflexes are generally normal

Clinical Characteristics of Primary Muscle Disease (Myopathy)

- Weakness, which usually affects proximal muscles, is present; weakness is usually slowly progressive but may be nonprogressive and asymmetric.
- Muscle atrophy may or may not be present.
- Weakness and atrophy are usually diffuse, particularly when the disease is established.
- Muscle tone is generally normal.
- Sensory reflexes are generally normal.

MOTOR NEURON DISEASE: AMYOTROPHIC LATERAL SCLEROSIS

- ALS is a progressive neuromuscular disorder caused by progressive degeneration or loss of motor neurons in the spinal cord, lower brain stem, nuclei, and motor cortex.
- The cause is unknown, but autoimmunity, viral infections, environmental factors (free radicals), and prions have been proposed as possibilities.
- Approximately 10% of cases are familial, and a defect in the superoxide dismutase gene (*SOD1*) has been recognized in familial cases.
- The incidence of ALS is approximately 2 in 100,000.
- Men are more often affected than women, and the peak age at onset is 40–50 years.

- The onset is usually insidious, with weakness and atrophy of distal muscles (e.g., hand muscles) that begin asymmetrically. The course in most cases is rapidly progressive, resulting in death from pulmonary infection within 3 years.

Diagnosis

The diagnosis of ALS is based on the clinical presentation and findings. The most useful confirmatory tests are NCSs and needle EMG. NCSs are usually within normal range, but needle EMG shows active and chronic neurogenic changes, which should be present in at least three limbs (tongue or paraspinal muscles may count as one limb). All patients with ALS should have NCSs, EMG, magnetic resonance imaging of the cervical region, heavy metal screening, serum protein electrophoresis, and measurement of parathyroid hormone level. Further testing is performed to exclude mimicking disorders.

Clinical Pearls

- Suspect ALS when a patient has a combination of upper motor neuron (weakness, spasticity, hyperreflexia, extensor plantar response, pseudobulbar) and lower motor neuron (weakness, atrophy, fasciculation) signs in more than two limbs (bulbar and/or paraspinal muscles are considered one limb).

- The following symptoms and signs are generally ***absent*** in ALS: extraocular muscle dysfunction, sensory and autonomic dysfunction, bladder dysfunction, and decline of cognition. If the patient presents initially with these symptoms and signs or if they constitute main features of the patient's problem, doubt the diagnosis of ALS.

Therapy

- Establish the diagnosis.
- Provide adequate information to the patient and/or care giver.
- Treatment is mostly supportive and symptomatic (i.e., in response to spasticity, cramps, depression, and pseudobulbar features).
- Currently, one drug has been approved by the U.S. Food and Drug Administration for treatment of ALS—riluzole (Rilutek), which may slow progression of the disease (50 mg bid orally). Trials of numerous other drugs are under way.
- Dysphagia is best managed by placement of a gastric tube and balanced nutrition.
- Respiratory failure may require mechanical support depending on the patient's wishes.

PERIPHERAL NEUROPATHIES

The approach to the evaluation of peripheral neuropathies is discussed in Chapter 16. This section discusses selected topics in neuropathy.

Common Mononeuropathies

Bell's Palsy

- Bell's palsy is also known as *acute idiopathic peripheral seventh nerve palsy*.
- The presentation is often unilateral, causing weakness of the facial muscles (forehead and lower face) manifested as difficulty in closing the eyes, wrinkling the forehead, smiling, or drinking.
- The cause is unknown, but postviral inflammation and autoimmunity have been proposed.
- The prognosis is worse when the weakness is severe or the proximal nerve is involved, manifesting as hyperacusis and decreased tearing or taste.

Diagnostic Testing
Most neurologists obtain a CBC, ESR, major component of adult hemoglobin C, thyroid function test, and angiotensin-converting enzyme level. NCSs and EMG may help to prognosticate (i.e., a decreasing amplitude of

action potential and denervation potentials in the facial muscles indicate a worse prognosis).

Differential Diagnosis
The differential diagnosis of Bell's palsy includes central seventh nerve palsy, often associated with an ipsilateral appendicular motor or sensory deficit. Cerebellopontine angle lesions often are associated with involvement of the fifth, sixth, and eighth nerves.

Treatment
Most neurologists administer a 7- to 10-day course of a corticosteroid (start at 60 mg/day) in the acute stage (within 5–7 days). Protect against corneal dryness and subsequent infection by patching the eye and administering artificial tears. The prognosis in Bell's palsy is generally favorable, with good recovery in up to 70% of cases. Patients should know this fact and also that the facial paralysis is not due to stroke.

Carpal Tunnel Syndrome

- Carpal tunnel syndrome, resulting from median nerve compression at the wrist, is the most common mononeuropathy and probably the most common cause of numbness of the hand.
- It presents with paresthesia and pain in the hand and arm that is usually worse at night and is relieved by rubbing or shaking the hand. In the chronic stage, weakness and atrophy of the thenar muscle may be seen.

- A positive Tinel's or Phalen's sign supports the diagnosis.

Evaluation
Patients with suspected carpal tunnel syndrome should be evaluated with a CBC, ESR, thyroid function test, and serum protein electrophoresis. The diagnosis is established by NCSs, which show delayed distal motor and sensory latency of the median nerve but relatively normal ulnar nerve latencies and conduction velocities.

Treatment
Treatment may be conservative (wrist splint) or symptomatic (pain medications). Short-term oral corticosteroid therapy may be given (prednisone, 60 mg/day tapering for 10 days). Local injection of corticosteroid into the wrist is usually not helpful. Other nonsurgical techniques include magnetic stimulation, but further study of the effectiveness of this therapy should be performed. The most effective therapy is surgical decompression of the nerve.

Cubital Tunnel Syndrome

- Cubital tunnel syndrome results from ulnar nerve compression at the elbow.
- The patient experiences usually bilateral numbness and paresthesia of the fourth and fifth fingers, followed by weakness and atrophy of the ulnar-innervated muscles of the hand. Pain is less common.

- The cause is unknown but could be related to repeated trauma to the elbow. Cubital tunnel syndrome must be differentiated from lower trunk plexus lesion (always look at the pupils for Horner's syndrome to rule out the possibility of an upper lobe tumor of the lung) and C7–8 radiculopathy.

Footdrop: Peroneal Nerve Palsy

- Peroneal nerve palsy results from compression of the peroneal nerve at the fibular head.
- The onset of the disease is usually acute. Predisposing factors include generalized neuropathy, crossing the legs for a long time, general anesthesia, weight loss, coma, and a knee cast.
- On examination, there is weakness of the foot dorsi- flexors and evertors. The patient is unable to stand or walk on the heels and has a steppage gait.
- Sensory complaints and deficits are minimal, and there are no reflex changes.
- Peroneal palsy must be differentiated from an L5 root lesion. In an L5 root lesion, often there is a history of back and radicular pain, weakness of the dorsiexten- sors and invertors of the foot, and weakness of the extensor hallucis longus. Knee jerk is diminished with an L5 root lesion. L5 radiculopathy is further differen- tiated from peroneal palsy by NCSs or EMG testing.

- Treatment is supportive—physical therapy and a short leg brace to improve walking by stabilizing the ankle joint.

Diabetic Neuropathies

Diabetes is the most common cause of polyneuropathy in Western countries. Its clinical presentations include

- Distal, symmetric sensory motor polyneuropathy
- Distal, symmetric sensory polyneuropathy
- Autonomic neuropathy: postural hypotension, dizziness, impotence, dry eyes or mouth, persistent diarrhea or nausea, bladder dysfunction
- Diabetic ophthalmoplegia: third nerve, often unilateral, pupillary response and size is usually normal
- Peripheral seventh nerve palsy
- Entrapment neuropathies: carpal and cubital tunnel syndromes, femoral neuropathy
- Thoracolumbar polyradiculopathy: must be differentiated from cardiopulmonary pathologies, acute abdominal pathology, and lumbar radiculopathy
- Diabetic amyotrophy: acute or subacute onset of thigh pain followed by weakness and later wasting of thigh and hip muscles (pelvifemoral distribution). The prognosis is generally good. Differential diagnosis includes lumbosacral polyradiculopathy, focal myositis, inclusion-body myositis, and femoral neuropathy

Hereditary Neuropathies:
Charcot-Marie-Tooth Disease

- Charcot-Marie-Tooth disease (CMT) is the most common inherited (autosomal dominant) polyneuropathy in humans.
- The prevalence is approximately 1 in 2,500.
- CMT-1 is referred to as hereditary motor sensory neuropathy (HMSN) type I, which is a demyelinating form, and CMT-2 (HMSN type II), which is a neuronal form affecting the dorsal root ganglion and lower motor neurons.
- CMT-1 is characterized by peroneal muscle atrophy, producing "stork legs" or legs with reverse champagne bottle appearance. Sensory impairment, pes cavus, hammer toe deformity, and hypertrophic nerves may also be seen. NCSs show marked decreased conduction velocities, decreased amplitude, and prolonged distal latencies. Nerve biopsy shows characteristics of onion-bulb formation, which reflects proliferation of Schwann cells, with demyelination and remyelination.
- In CMT-2, NCSs show only slightly slowed conduction velocities, and nerve biopsy shows axonal degeneration and regeneration.
- Other inherited neuropathies include
  - HMSN III (also known as *Dejerine-Sottas* or *CMT-3*), which starts in childhood and progresses to severe

disability (patients are wheelchair bound in their teens). NCSs show marked slowing of conduction velocities (<10 m/sec).

- Hereditary neuropathy with liability to pressure palsy: autosomal dominant, presents with mononeuropathy multiplex and multiple pressure palsies (often due to minor pressure). NCSs show demyelinating neuropathy with features of compression (delayed distal motor and sensory latencies). Nerve biopsy shows focal demyelination and remyelination producing sausagelike "tomaculous" structures on tease nerve fiber preparation.
- DNA testing is now commercially available for diagnosis of CMT-1 and CMT-3, which shows duplication at chromosome 17 P11-2 and deletion in hereditary neuropathy with liability to pressure palsy.

DISORDERS OF THE NEUROMUSCULAR JUNCTION

Postsynaptic Disorders: Acquired Myasthenia Gravis

- Myasthenia gravis (MG) is the most well-known autoimmune disease in humans.
- The disease is caused by an immune attack against the postsynaptic (end-plate) membrane of the neuromuscular junction of the skeletal muscle.

- The onset is often acute or subacute and may be triggered by stress, infection, surgery, pregnancy, drugs, and other unknown environmental factors.
- The disease has two peak onsets of age: 20–30 years of age in women and 50–60 years in men.
- The clinical hallmarks of MG are fluctuating muscle weakness and fatigue. The most typical presentation is weakness in the distribution of the ocular (ptosis, diplopia) and bulbar muscles (dysphasia, dysphonia, and dysarthria). The limb muscles are less affected. Onset of MG with proximal limb and respiratory muscle weakness is rare.
- Muscle tone, bulk, sensory function, and reflexes are otherwise normal unless the patient has other medical and neurologic diseases.

Diagnosis

Diagnosis of MG is made on the basis of the typical clinical features and is confirmed further by the following:

   1. *Edrophonium (Tensilon) test.* The Tensilon test is a quick and easy test for diagnosing MG. The Tensilon dose is 10 mg (1 ml), given intravenously (IV). Before performing the Tensilon test, establish muscle weakness that can be measured objectively (ptosis, diplopia, dysarthria). If there is no good objective weakness, in my experience the test is unreliable and not helpful. Administer 2 mg as a test dose and monitor heart rate (pulse)

and blood pressure. If no reaction is seen, give another 3 mg; if no response is seen, administer the remaining 5 mg. The response should be dramatic and objective to be considered positive. Always have a vial of atropine on the side to overcome excessive muscarinic side effects. Tensilon acts quickly, and the response may last 10–15 minutes. Elderly patients with asthma or chronic obstructive pulmonary disease and cardiac disease are best monitored carefully in the hospital; otherwise, the Tensilon test may be done in the office. An unequivocally positive Tensilon test is diagnostic for the typical presentation of MG. Remember that Tensilon may improve fatigue in many neuromuscular diseases, but the response usually is not as dramatic as in MG.

2. *Electrophysiologic tests.* NCSs and needle EMG results are usually normal in patients with MG but need to be done to exclude other neuromuscular diseases. Two electrophysiologic tests are done for confirmation of neuromuscular junction disease:

- **Repetitive nerve stimulation (Jolly test).** A gradual decreasing amplitude of motor nerve action potential (decremental response) of the muscle is seen when the innervated nerve is stimulated at a rate of 2 per second (up to 10% decrement is normal). The sensitivity of this test is approximately 60%.
- **Single-fiber EMG.** This test is a more complex and highly sensitive test in which the time interval between two muscle fibers belonging to one ante-

rior horn cell is measured by a special needle electrode. The two muscle fibers usually fire simultaneously, with minimal contraction of the muscle, but in MG they do not fire simultaneously (increased variability or jitter). Single-fiber EMG is highly sensitive (i.e., a weak muscle due to MG is always abnormal) but is highly nonspecific (i.e., results are abnormal in many neuromuscular diseases).

3. ***Acetylcholine receptor antibody.*** This test is highly specific for MG (very rarely reported in other conditions). More than 90% of patients with moderately severe generalized MG test positive for the antibody, but in purely ocular MG the results are positive in approximately 50% of patients. Approximately 10% of patients with generalized MG have negative antibody tests results.

4. ***Other autoantibodies.*** Tests for antistriate muscle antibody and anticitric acid antibody are useful in patients suspected of having thymoma (elderly patients). Remember that not all enlarged thymus glands on chest CT scan have positive antistriate muscle antibody, and tests for the antibody are not always negative in patients with a small thymus gland. The value of this antibody test is that if the test and chest CT scan are both negative for thymoma, thymectomy is not necessary in an elderly patient, and if the test is positive, thymectomy may be considered if the patient is medically stable.

5. ***Other blood tests***: ESR, antinuclear antibody, serum CK, thyroid function test, and rheumatoid factor.

6. ***Imaging.*** Routine chest x-ray is indicated in suspected adult-onset MG. An elderly patient needs chest CT to rule out thymoma.

Treatment

Symptomatic Treatment

The symptoms of MG may be treated with **acetylcholinesterase (AChE) inhibitors.** The most commonly used drug is pyridostigmine (Mestinon) given orally (60-mg tablets). Start at a low dose and titrate according to response. The side effects should be explained to the patient. Overmedication with Mestinon may exacerbate weakness (cholinergic crisis). The IV dose of Mestinon is 2 mg (equal to 60 mg orally).

Immunosuppressive Therapy

Immunosuppressive therapy for MG includes

- Corticosteroids
- Immunosuppressive drugs: azathioprine, cyclophosphamide, cyclosporine-A, methotrexate
- Thymectomy: trans-sternal or maximal (trans-sternal + transcervical)
- Immunomodulating agents: not widely used
- Plasmapheresis (plasma exchange): for acute worsening of MG (e.g., crisis, post-thymectomy)
- Intravenous immunoglobulin (IVIG): for acute weakness

Guidelines for Therapy

1. Establish the diagnosis of MG before initiating therapy.
2. Individualize the therapeutic choices.
3. Explain the advantages and disadvantages of each therapeutic option to the patient.
4. The goal of therapy is to achieve clinical remission (no fatigable muscle or weakness without receiving any medications).
5. Titrate the dose of the AChE inhibitor according to the patient's response to achieve the optimal response. If the patient does not respond to an adequate dose (240 mg/day for most patients), increasing the dose not only does not help but also can cause side effects and exacerbate weakness. AChE inhibitors are good for symptomatic relief; if they do not help strength, there is no point in using them or increasing the dose.
6. Thymectomy is indicated in all patients aged 15–60 years with stable medical conditions. Patients with thymoma should have thymectomy regardless of age. Most neurologists do not recommend thymectomy for pure ocular MG.
7. Most centers do trans-sternal thymectomy. Thymectomy should be done in a center with experienced surgeons and a team knowledgeable about the disease.

8. Thymectomy is an elective surgery and should not be done urgently. Patients should be stabilized and as strong as possible before thymectomy. The response to thymectomy is often delayed (up to 2 years on average). The advantage of thymectomy is the long-term benefit of an increased chance of achieving long-lasting remission. In general, early thymectomy is recommended (after adequate stabilization).

9. Corticosteroids are given to patients with a suboptimal response to AChE inhibitors or who worsen post-thymectomy. In patients with more severe MG, begin with a high daily dose of prednisone (e.g., 60 mg/day) and continue to reach a maximum response (usually takes 3–4 weeks). Then change to a high alternate daily dose (e.g., 110 mg qod) and continue another 2–3 weeks before you begin slow tapering. If you choose to give a high daily dose, it is advisable to hospitalize the patient in case the patient's condition worsens. In patients with milder cases, you may begin with a low alternate dose (20 mg qod) with gradual incremental increases. This can be done on an outpatient basis. Some patients with ocular MG may require prednisone therapy.

10. Immunosuppressive drugs (e.g., azathioprine) are given to patients who develop undesirable side effects to prednisone, cannot take corticosteroids, or have a relapse when prednisone is tapered.

Immunosuppressive drugs act slowly, and their side effects should be monitored closely. Most neurologists use azathioprine (Imuran), 150–200 mg per day.

11. Plasma exchange (plasmapheresis) is usually considered for acute exacerbation of MG (myasthenic crisis, post-thymectomy worsening), and some authorities use exchange before thymectomy. The results of plasma exchange are fast (usually after the second or third exchange), but its effect is short lived (3 months at most). It is considered a quick booster. Exchange has a medium morbidity rate and is a costly procedure.

12. IVIG: The indications and costs are the same as for plasma exchange, but it is easier to use and is more available. Therapeutic responses to it are unpredictable, however.

Clinical Pearls

- Suspect MG in young adults presenting with new onset of diplopia or ptosis. Doubt MG when a patient presents with generalized fatigue without fluctuation and absence of ocular or bulbar muscle dysfunction after 2–3 years.
- The hallmark of muscle weakness in MG is its fluctuation (variable, worse on exertion and better after rest)

and the distribution of affected muscles (ocular or bulbar and extremities).

- Always obtain an adequate history of prescribed medication, because some drugs can produce myasthenic features (e.g., mycin antibiotics, antiepileptic drugs, antiarrhythmics, penicillamine).
- Establish muscle weakness objectively before doing a Tensilon test.
- The sensitivity of repetitive nerves will increase if several muscles are tested.
- The most specific and sensitive test for diagnosis of MG is acetylcholine receptor antibody, but it should be performed in a reliable laboratory.
- Chest x-ray and CT scan are indicated in all myasthenic patients.
- The goal of therapy is to achieve remission without medication or with very low doses of medication.
- Individualize therapeutic choices because not only are patients with MG different individuals but also their disease presentations are different and even degree of muscle weakness is different from muscle to muscle in a given patient.
- Thymectomy is an elective surgery and should not be done urgently when the patient is weak or unstable. Thymectomy should be done in a center with experienced surgeons and neurologists.

Presynaptic Disorders

Lambert-Eaton Myasthenic Syndrome

Lambert-Eaton myasthenic syndrome (LEMS) is a slowly progressive, proximal (hip and shoulder girdle) weakness.

Clinical Features

- Ocular, bulbar, and respiratory muscles are usually spared or less affected.
- Autonomic symptoms such as dry mouth, constipation, and impotence are common.
- **Hint:** Always consider LEMS when an elderly patient presents with weakness and a dry mouth.
- Reflexes are generally depressed.
- Muscle strength and reflexes may enhance transiently with exercise (i.e., warm up).
- LEMS is associated with underlying malignancy in approximately 60% of elderly patients with LEMS (small cell carcinoma of the lung is the most common).
- The majority of patients with LEMS have an antibody against the N and L types of voltage-gated calcium channels in the presynaptic membrane. The antibody can be detected in the serum of 60% of patients.

Diagnostic Tests

- Male patients should have a test for antineuronal antibody (anti-Hu), a chest CT scan, bronchoscopy, and other tests for detecting underlying carcinoma.

- Diagnosis of LEMS is best confirmed by electrophysiologic testing. The most characteristic result is decreased amplitude of the muscle action potential at baseline. Repetitive nerve stimulation at slow-rate stimulation (2 per second) shows decremental response, but in contrast to MG, a higher rate of stimulation (e.g., 20 per second) or stimulation after brief exercise (10 seconds) of the muscle shows marked increasing of the amplitude (incremental responses). This marked increase after brief exercise is the most common characteristic of LEMS and other presynaptic disorders. Single-fiber EMG shows significant increase of "jitter" value, as seen in MG.

Treatment

- In LEMS, any underlying carcinoma should be treated.
- AChE inhibitors may help some patients.
- 3',4'-diaminopyridine is probably the most effective drug for symptomatic relief but has not yet been approved by the U.S. Food and Drug Administration. This drug blocks outward potassium current, which prolongs the duration of activation of acetylcholine in the presynaptic membrane and increases calcium entry to preterminal membrane and further release of acetylcholine. The drug also helps autonomic symptoms. The dose is 15–60 mg qid. A higher dose may result in cardiac arrhythmia and seizure.

Botulism

Botulism is caused by ingestion of a neurotoxin (type A, B, or E) produced by anaerobic gram-negative *Clostridium botulinum*, often from improperly canned foods (home canned, home-processed, low-acid foods) or through wounds and possibly IV drug abuse.

Clinical Features
Botulism presents with sudden onset of blurred vision, diplopia, bulbar dysfunction (dysarthria, dysphagia), and symmetric, descending limb weakness. Autonomic symptoms such as dry mouth and dilated, fixed pupils may be seen.

Diagnostic Tests
The diagnosis is confirmed by repetitive nerve stimulants showing incremental response (similar to that in LEMS). Further evaluation includes head CT scan and lumbar puncture to exclude mimicking disorders. More specific tests for botulism are the mouse inoculation test for toxin and serum and stool or food cultures for detecting the organism. The differential diagnosis includes MG and Guillain-Barré syndrome (Miller-Fisher variant).

Treatment
Treatment includes ventilatory support, AChE inhibitors, and trivalent equine antitoxin, which can be life saving if used early.

MUSCLE DISEASES (MYOPATHIES)

Inflammatory Myopathies

The inflammatory myopathies include polymyositis (PM), dermatomyositis (DM), and inclusion body myositis (IBM).

Polymyositis

- The onset of PM may be acute or subacute, with symmetric proximal muscle weakness (difficulty rising from a chair or combing hair).
- Muscle tone and bulk are normal at the onset.
- Sensory examination and reflexes are normal, and muscle pain occurs in only one-third of patients.
- Most patients with PM have joint pain and dysphagia.
- PM rarely affects children younger than age 15.
- The disease is caused by an autoimmune attack against the muscle fibers. It may be associated with other autoimmune diseases (overlap syndrome).
- Serum CK concentration is often moderately elevated.
- NCSs are normal; however, needle EMG shows spontaneous potentials in the form of fibrillation, positive sharp waves, and small, polyphasic short-duration, low-amplitude motor unit potentials.
- The diagnosis is confirmed by muscle biopsy, which shows muscle fiber necrosis, regeneration, and inflammatory cell infiltrate around and invading the muscle

fibers. Because of sampling error, negative biopsy does not rule out the diagnosis.

- Treatment is with corticosteroids, immunosuppressive drugs, and IVIG. In intractable cases, plasma exchange or total body irradiation may be considered.

Dermatomyositis

- Patients with DM experience mild, proximal muscle weakness.
- Skin lesions are characteristic: heliotropic rashes around the eye and over the cheeks, sternum, and overextensors of the joint. **Gottren's papules**—scaly, violet rashes over the knuckles—are diagnostic. DM is not simply PM with a skin lesion; it is a separate inflammatory myopathy. Nailbed telangiectasia and necrosis may be seen. Unlike PM, DM can affect children.
- Serum CK concentration may be mild to moderately elevated.
- EMG shows myopathic features as in PM.
- DM is highly associated with other autoimmune diseases.
- Association with malignancy is approximately 10%, particularly in elderly patients. Patients with late-onset DM should be evaluated for malignancy.
- Autoantibodies associated with DM include anti PM-1, anti JO-1, and anti-Ro. They are not only associated with overlap syndrome but also indicate cardiomy-

opathy or interstitial lung disease associated with DM or PM.

- The diagnosis is confirmed by muscle biopsy, which typically shows inflammatory cells around the blood vessel wall (vasculitis). Immune deposits may be demonstrated in the endothelial membrane. The hallmark of muscle biopsy, however, is atrophy of the muscle fibers at the periphery of the muscle fascicle (***perifascicular atrophy***).
- Treatment of DM is the same as that for PM.

Inclusion Body Myositis

- IBM (sporadic form) is a disease of the elderly, with onset at age 50 years or older.
- The muscle weakness affects not only proximal muscles but also distal muscles. The distribution of weakness may be symmetric or asymmetric.
- Serum CK concentration is mildly elevated.
- IBM is usually not associated with malignancy or other autoimmune diseases.
- The results of EMG show mixed myopathic and neurogenic changes.
- The cause is unknown but an autoimmune theory is the strongest.
- The diagnosis is confirmed by muscle biopsy, which shows muscle necrosis and a mild to moderate inflammatory response. The most characteristic result is the presence of rimmed vacuoles that contain filamentous

inclusions demonstrated by electron microscopy. Remember that rimmed vacuoles are also seen in other myopathies. If the clinical presentation is typical, the presence of rimmed vacuoles may be diagnostic.

- **Caveat:** In practice, IBM probably is more common than PM or DM. Suspect IBM when an elderly patient has weakness in the proximal and distal muscles and in evaluation you find mildly elevated serum CK concentration and mixed neurogenic-myopathic results on EMG. Consider muscle biopsy in these patients. Also suspect IBM when a patient with a previous diagnosis of PM does not respond to corticosteroids or immunosuppressive drugs, and consider repeating muscle biopsy.

There is no effective treatment available for IBM, but most neurologists consider a trial of immunosuppressive drugs or corticosteroids for 6 months to 1 year. Use of IVIG has shown promise in some patients.

Congenital Myopathies

- Congenital myopathies are a slowly progressive or nonprogressive group of muscle diseases.
- The onset is usually in childhood, but adult onset may be seen.
- Clinically, patients exhibit ocular or proximal muscle weakness.
- Reflexes may be normal or depressed.

- Dysmorphic features (bone, joint) are common.
- NCSs and needle EMG may be normal or show a mixed myopathic-neurogenic pattern.
- Serum CK concentration may be normal or mildly elevated.
- Diagnosis is confirmed by muscle biopsy, which shows myopathic features and specific structural changes in the muscle fibers for which the name of myopathy is given: central core disease, nemaline (rod) myopathy, and centronuclear (myotubular) myopathy.

Muscular Dystrophies

- Muscular dystrophies are hereditary, progressive myopathies with onset of muscle weakness in early childhood or adulthood.
- Muscle atrophy is usually seen.
- Their names indicate that they are due to a deficiency of protein (dystrophin), as in Duchenne's muscular dystrophy and Becker's muscular dystrophy, or that they have unique clinical features, such as fascioscapulohumeral (FSH) muscular dystrophy, myotonic muscular dystrophy, scapuloperoneal muscular dystrophy, Emery-Dreifuss muscular dystrophy, and limb girdle muscular dystrophy.
- The diagnosis is confirmed by elevated serum CK concentration, DNA analysis, and muscle biopsy.

Myotonic Muscular Dystrophy

- Myotonic muscular dystrophy is the most common muscular dystrophy in adults, with a prevalence of 1 in 8,000.
- It has autosomal dominant inheritance.
- The gene defect is located in the long arm of chromosome 19, and the severity of disease increases with successive generations (known as *anticipation*).
- The clinical manifestations vary from patient to patient and even among siblings.
- It is a multiple-system disease: muscle, heart, gastrointestinal (GI) tract, endocrine system, skin, and brain are affected.
- Muscle weakness and atrophy affect the distal muscles more than the proximal. Typical features include temporalis muscle atrophy, bifacial diplegia, bilateral ptosis, weakness and atrophy of the sternocleidomastoid muscles, atrophy of the forearm muscles, and weakness of the wrist extensors and feet dorsiflexors.
- Reflexes are depressed or absent.
- The characteristic myotonia (delayed muscle relaxation) is seen in the hand grip ("grip myotonia" or "prolonged handshake sign") and percussion myotonia (myotonia induced by tapping the muscle).
- Dysarthria and dysphagia are seen in the advanced stage.
- Systemic signs include frontal baldness, cataract, cardiac conduction defect, GI dysfunction, testicular

atrophy, diabetes, mental retardation, and sleep apnea syndrome.

- The diagnosis is based on clinical features (phenotype) and confirmed by DNA analysis, which shows expansion of the trinucleotide repeat (known as *CTG repeat*). A normal repeat is 5–30; more than 50 is abnormal. The longer the repeat, the worse the disease is and the longer the duration of the disease will be. All patients should have CTG analysis, cardiac evaluation, and slit-lamp examination.
- EMG shows a typical "dive bomber" sound or myotonic discharge on needle examination and myopathic features.
- Therapy is supportive. Antimyotonic drugs include phenytoin, procainamide, mexiletine, acetazolamide, and dantrolene.

Fascioscapulohumeral Muscular Dystrophy

- FSH muscular distropy is the second most common muscular dystrophy in adults.
- The prevalence is approximately 1 in 20,000.
- Onset is usually in midadulthood, with weakness of the facial muscles (difficulty in drinking with a straw, whistling, and smiling) and later weakness and atrophy of the scapular fixator, neck extensors, biceps, and foot dorsiflexors. Prominent winging of the scapula, "Pop-eye" appearance of the arm, and pectoralis muscle crease are unique clinical features.

- The defect is at the 4q35 location in chromosome 4. DNA analysis demonstrates deletion at 4q35 in sporadic cases.
- Severity varies among affected family members.
- Muscle biopsy shows myopathic features and inflammatory response in 20–30% of cases.
- Serum CK concentration is mildly elevated, and EMG shows myopathic features.
- Treatment is supportive and symptomatic.

Metabolic Myopathies

Primary

Primary metabolic myopathies include disorders of carbohydrate metabolism (McArdle's [myophosphorylase deficiency], phosphofructokinase deficiency, and acid maltase deficiency), disorders of lipid metabolism (carnitine deficiency and carnitine palmitoyl transferase deficiency), mitochondrial myopathies, and other myopathies such as myoadenylate deaminase deficiency.

Secondary

Secondary metabolic myopathies include myopathies caused by an endocrine disorder or and toxic or drug-induced myopathies.

Metabolic myopathies generally present with muscle pain, cramps, and weakness, and sometimes with episodes of myoglobinuria and lactic acidosis. Some are genetically determined. Diagnosis is made on the basis of clinical presentation, serum CK level, myoglobinuria, abnormal exercise test response, muscle biopsy, and DNA analysis. Treatment is supportive and symptomatic, and enzyme replacement may help. Patients with mitochondrial myopathies may be helped by administration of vitamins C, K, and B complex and coenzyme Q10.

20

Back and Neck Pain

Back and neck pain are common complaints and are the
main reasons for work-related injury and disability claims.
Many conditions cause back and neck pain (e.g., spinal,
nonspinal, psychological).

MUSCLE SPRAIN

Muscle sprain or strain commonly occurs after minor
trauma, causing shearing of muscle and fascia. Sprains
present with localized, constant, deep pain without radiation to the limb. There are no neurologic symptoms. Treatment is symptomatic, and no diagnostic testing is
necessary.

RADICULOPATHIES

A spinal root can be compressed by any lesion; the two
leading causes are herniated nuclear pulposus and
spondylosis. Radiculopathy typically presents with back or
neck pain that radiates to the limb in a distribution corresponding to that of the compressed nerve root. Pain is
usually dull and achy but may be sharp. The pain is aggra-

vated by walking, standing, twisting, bending, sneezing, coughing, or straining. Pain may be relieved by rest or knee or hip flexion. The onset of radiculopathy can be spontaneous but usually starts after minor trauma, lifting heavy objects, or repeated bending. Some patients may complain of sensory symptoms such as paresthesia or limb weakness (foot dragging, footdrop). The common root syndromes in the back are S1 root due to herniated L5–S1, intervertebral disk, and L5 root caused by disk herniation of L4–5 interspace. In cervical regions, C6 and C7 root compressions are the two most common root syndromes. Memorize the myotome and dermatome distribution of these four common root syndromes. Remember that the L5 root has no reflex level. Knee jerk is for the L4 root and ankle jerk is for the S1 root. Footdrop can be seen in L5 root lesion, but if the tibialis anterior muscle is innervated by L4 (which is normally seen in some individuals), footdrop may not occur.

Caveat: An elderly patient who has spontaneous onset of low back pain with or without root symptoms should be considered to have spinal metastasis until proved otherwise. In the lumbosacral region, disk herniation compresses the root laterally, but in the cervical region, the disk may compress the root laterally and spinal cord posteriorly (myelopathy). Central disk herniation or spondylosis can compress multiple lumbosacral roots and present with cauda equina or conus medullaris syndrome, which are neurologic urgencies.

LUMBAR STENOSIS

Lumbar stenosis is caused by slowly progressive hypertrophy of the vertebral facets and degeneration of the vertebrae and disks, causing narrowing of the nerve root foramina and spinal canal. This condition is common in elderly individuals and presents with symptoms and signs referable to bilateral lumbosacral polyradiculopathy. Most patients complain of dull, constant back pain and sometimes paresthesia of the lower extremities, which are aggravated by walking or standing (spinal or neurogenic claudication) and relieved by stooping or sitting down. Nonsteroidal anti-inflammatory drugs and physical therapy help the pain in most patients.

EVALUATION

History

In evaluating back and neck pain, the history should include

- Onset and location of pain
- Aggravating and relieving factors
- What caused the pain: accident, lifting, bending, or spontaneous
- Any complaints about weakness or sensory symptoms
- Any bowel or bladder dysfunction
- History of claudication

- Question: Does position or movement of the limb affect the pain?

General Physical Examination

1. Examine the spine for any deformity or curvature.
2. Test the spine for range of motion.
3. Check the spine for focal tenderness and paraspinal muscle spasm.
4. Examine the gait.
5. Do a straight leg raising test in lumbosacral radiculopathy.
6. Do Patrick's test if sacroiliac osteoarthritis is suspected.
7. Examine the abdomen and take pelvic or peripheral pulses in an atypical presentation.

Focused Neurologic Examination

Perform a focused neurologic examination taking the following steps to establish objective evidence of **spinal nerve root or spinal cord compression**:

1. Examine strength and differentiate muscle weakness from weakness due to pain.
2. Test for dermatomal sensory loss.
3. Check for the presence or absence of reflexes.
4. Check muscle tone.
5. Assess gait.

6. Assess for the presence or absence of long tract signs (hyperreflexia, clonus, Babinski's sign).
7. In a patient with suspected cauda equina, check for saddle anesthesia, rectal tone, and anal wink reflex.

Clinical point: The history and examination of patients with back and neck pain should be directed toward finding an organic cause known as a "red flag," such as cancer, neurologic diseases, infection, or disk herniation.

Diagnostic Tests

The following tests aid in the diagnosis of back and neck pain:

- **Neuroimaging**, including plain x-ray, computed tomography and magnetic resonance imaging scans, and bone scans. The imaging technique should be selected on an individual basis; not all patients with neck or back pain need neuroimaging.
- **Nerve conduction studies and electromyography (EMG)** show the electrophysiologic changes of root compression. They are best performed 2–3 weeks after onset. Be specific when you are ordering the test. Patients with radiculopathy who do not respond initially to treatment or develop motor or sensory deficit need an EMG.
- **Blood tests:** erythrocyte sedimentation rate, serum protein electrophoresis, prostatic surface antigen, complete blood cell count, chemistry profile (in selected cases).

TREATMENT

Conservative and Medical Treatment

- Bed rest, avoidance of lifting, and weight reduction
- Neck traction, cervical collar, or back brace
- Analgesic (nonsteroidal anti-inflammatory drugs)
- Muscle relaxants: usually are not helpful
- Physical therapy and back exercises when acute pain has subsided

Surgical Procedures

Surgical procedures include laminectomy, diskectomy, and spinal fusion. Surgical intervention is considered in the following situations:

- Failed response to conservative and medical therapy
- Progressive neurologic deficit
- Cauda equina/conus medullaris syndromes
- Signs of cord compression
- Symptomatic spinal stenosis when it is resistant to medical and conservative treatment

Caveat: In acute lumbosacral radiculopathy, a few days of rest is adequate, particularly if the history is clear for acute radiculopathy (e.g., back pain after a heavy lift). No diagnostic testing is necessary at the beginning. Only 10% of patients with radiculopathy need surgery. Pain alone is not a good reason for surgery.

Neurologic Urgencies
and Emergencies

21

Coma

TERMINOLOGY

Coma: A state of unconsciousness and unresponsiveness to external stimuli.

Persistent vegetative state (PVS): Often occurs after coma. Patients appear to be conscious but are unaware of surroundings and self. The signs must persist at least 1 month before the diagnosis of PVS may be made.

Locked-in syndrome: Occurs commonly after surviving coma. Patients are quadriplegic but can communicate with eye or head movements.

Brain death: Comatose (due to an irreversible cause) and unresponsive to noxious stimuli. Cortical and brain stem reflexes are lost. May need further confirmation by absence of brain activity on electroencephalogram (EEG) or absence of cerebral blood flow on brain scan if clinical criteria are met for at least 6 hours. Confirmatory test is not required if duration is 12–24 hours.

COMA: A MEDICAL EMERGENCY

Coma is a medical emergency, requiring prompt diagnosis and management. The following steps should be taken:

1. Stabilize the patient first.
2. Obtain a history, and do a careful examination.
3. Do a quick neurologic examination appropriate for the comatose patient and interpret your findings.
4. Locate the site of the lesion, according to the physical and neurologic signs.
5. Try to discern the most likely cause or causes and remember that coma is a sign of underlying pathology. Remember the most common causes of coma are toxic and metabolic derangements, which are potentially treatable and reversible.
6. All patients should have head neuroimaging (computed tomography [CT] or magnetic resonance imaging [MRI]).
7. Try to prognosticate the outcome of the patient.

STABILIZING THE PATIENT

Take the following steps to stabilize the patient:

1. Clear the airway and intubate if necessary.
2. Oxygenate.
3. Maintain circulation.
4. Establish an intravenous (IV) line and draw blood for measurement of complete blood cell count,

chemistry profile, toxin-drug screening, antiepileptic drug levels, and arterial blood gases.
5. Administer 100 mg IV thiamine, 50 ml/50% dextrose (if fingerstick glucose <80 mg), and 2 mg naloxone hydrochloride (Narcan) if narcotic overdose is suspected. If bilateral small pupils do not dilate after 10 mg of Narcan, opiate intoxication may be ruled out.

Caveat: Patients with global ischemic-hypoxic encephalopathy (e.g., post–cardiac arrest) may not need glucose because further elevation of glucose may cause further neuronal damage.

HISTORY AND PHYSICAL EXAMINATION

Obtain history from relatives, friends, police, and paramedics. Witnesses should not leave the hospital until questioned thoroughly. Obtain medical, neurologic, and psychiatric histories. Establish the onset of coma (acute, subacute, or chronic).

Physical examination should begin with assessment of blood pressure, pulse, respiration, and temperature. Inspect the skin for needle tracks, jaundice, spider angiomata, petechiae, lacerations, hematoma, ecchymosis, bleeding, and fracture.

NEUROLOGIC EXAMINATION

Doing a complete neurologic examination in comatose patients is not only impractical but also unnecessary. However, most authorities recommend performing a limited neurologic examination as follows in all comatose patients:

A. **Look at the patient.** Note the following:
   1. Any movements
   2. Any abnormal movements (e.g., myoclonia, seizures, asterixis)
   3. Any asymmetry of limb position: paralysis
B. **Head and neck**
   1. Inspect head, neck, and face for signs of trauma; look for tongue lacerations (sign of seizures)
   2. Meningismus: subarachnoid hemorrhage (SAH), meningitis
      Caveat: In post-traumatic coma, do not manipulate the neck unless neck fracture or dislocation has been excluded by x-ray.
C. **Look at the patient's eyes.** In comatose patients, the eyes are closed due to tonic eyelid contraction. This also indicates the upper pons is intact. Remember that in the comatose patient, there is no resistance to passive eye opening. In psychogenic coma, there is resistance.

D. **Pupils**
1. Check the size: small, pinpoint, dilated, or normal
2. Check for symmetry: equal or asymmetric (anisocoria)
3. Check reaction to direct light: normal, sluggish, unreactive
   a. Bilateral, small, reactive: pontine lesion, toxic-metabolic
   b. Small, midsize, reactive: metabolic-toxic
   c. Bilateral, dilated, fixed (unreactive): severe anoxia, glutethimide and/or atropine poisoning
   d. Unequal, dilated: third nerve palsy, uncal herniation
   e. Unequal, small, fixed (reactive): Horner's syndrome, midbrain disease, thalamic disorder
      Caveats: Anisocoria in comatose patients should be considered pathologic until proved otherwise. Beware of eyedrops because they can affect pupillary responses. At times, it is necessary to use magnifying glasses to observe subtle pupillary responses. Spontaneous rhythmic pupillary contraction is called *hippus*. In general, reactive, symmetric pupils indicate a toxic-metabolic cause of coma, and unreactive, asymmetric pupils indicate a structural lesion.

E. **Eye movements**
   1. **Spontaneous.** Look at the eyes and note
      a. **Roving eye movements:** slow, horizontal, side-to-side eye movements: intact brain stem
      b. **Nystagmus:** posterior fossa lesion, drug intoxication (e.g., antiepileptic drug levels), seizures
      c. **Ocular bobbing:** slow upward and rapid downward movement seen commonly in pontine hemorrhage
      d. **Ocular dipping:** slow downward and rapid upward movement seen in pontine lesion
      e. **Conjugate eye deviation away from paretic side:** seen commonly in pontine lesion
      f. **Conjugate eye deviation toward paretic side:** supratentorial lesion stroke
      g. **Disconjugate eye deviation:** brain stem lesion
      h. **Skew deviation (one eye up and other down):** brain stem lesion, pontine tegmentum
      i. **Persistent downward gaze:** tectal lesion
      j. **Persistent upward gaze:** probable nonconvulsive status epilepticus
   2. **Reflexive**
      a. **Oculocephalic or "doll's eye" test:** In a comatose patient with intact brain stem, brisk lateral head movements cause the eyes to move contralaterally.

Caveats: Do not perform this maneuver in a patient in post-traumatic coma unless neck injury has already been ruled out. Do not do this maneuver briskly in elderly patients.

b. **Oculovestibular** (caloric test): To test lateral eye movements, first check the ears to rule out bleeding or a perforated tympanic membrane. The ear canal should be clean. Elevate the head 30 degrees. Irrigate one ear at a time. In the comatose patient with an intact brain stem, ice-cold water (10–20°C) causes the eyes to move slowly (tonically) toward the side of irrigation. Try more water if there is no response (sometimes 200 ml is necessary). Irrigate the other ear after 10 minutes. To evaluate vertical eye movements, irrigate both ears simultaneously (cold = downward; warm = upward). Remember that in a conscious person, unilateral ice-cold water irrigation moves the eyes toward the side of stimulation but causes nystagmus to the opposite direction; with warm water irrigation, the nystagmus is toward the side of stimulation.

F. **Motor response**
  1. Look for spontaneous limb movements: Diminishment of movement on one side suggests a structural lesion.

2. If there are no spontaneous limb movements, try to induce movements with noxious stimuli and note whether movement is purposeful, unilateral (structural lesion), or absent (poor prognosis, but beware of quadriplegia due to spinal cord lesions, acute neuropathy, locked-in syndrome, or use of paralyzing agents).

G. **Abnormal postures**
   1. **Decorticate** or flexor posture: bilateral hemispheric lesions, bilateral internal capsule insults, or thalamic lesions
   2. **Decerebrate** or extensor posture: brain stem lesion or metabolic derangement
   3. **Diagonal** posture: decorticate on one side and decerebrate on the opposite; supratentorial lesion or lesion at the level of the vestibular nuclei

H. **Respiratory pattern.** Note the respiratory pattern if the patient is not intubated and ventilated mechanically.
   1. **Normal pattern:** metabolic causes
   2. **Cheyne-Stokes:** metabolic, hypoxic, diffuse bihemispheric
   3. **Ataxic:** very irregular; brain stem lesion, particularly medullary lesion; also seen in meningitis
   4 **Apneustic:** prolonged inspiration or expiration; midpons lesion

5. **Hypoventilation:** metabolic, increased intracranial pressure (ICP), drug overdose (sedative-hypnotic)
6. **Hyperventilation:** metabolic, brain stem lesion
   Caveat: If the patient has ataxic respiration, use of a sedative drug may cause respiratory arrest.

I. **Other neurologic signs**
   1. Muscle stretch reflexes are not helpful in evaluation of coma, because they may be preserved despite severe brain insult. Asymmetry of reflexes, however, can be useful.
   2. Long tract signs, such as spasticity and pathologic reflexes (Babinski's sign), commonly indicate a structural lesion.
   3. Bilateral papilledema indicates increased ICP but may be seen a few days after onset of coma.

DIFFERENTIAL DIAGNOSIS

Combine the history, physical examination, and neurologic findings and note the following clues:

- Gradual onset of coma, without clear-cut focal or lateralizing signs and preserved pupillary reflex, is seen commonly in toxic-metabolic disorders.
- Meningeal signs, with or without fever and with or without lateralizing signs, raise the possibility of SAH. **Caveat:** In profound coma, neck stiffness may be absent.

- Sudden onset of coma with focal or lateralizing neurologic signs and abnormal pupillary responses or eye movement abnormalities indicates subtentorial lesion (posterior fossa and brain stem).
- Gradual onset of coma with rostrocaudal deterioration, associated with lateralizing neurologic deficit with or without pupillary abnormalities and eye movement abnormalities, indicates supratentorial lesions, such as massive stroke or hemorrhage.

SPECIFIC LABORATORY STUDIES

- CT or MRI scans of the head are indicated for all patients in coma without obvious cause to assess the nature and severity of the structural lesion.
- An EEG also is recommended for all comatose patients to assess the cause (toxic-metabolic encephalopathy), assess seizures, and help in determining the prognosis.
- X-ray of the cervical spine is indicated in all cases of traumatic coma.
- Lumbar puncture is recommended when SAH or meningitis is suspected.

PROGNOSIS

Generally, the prognosis for the coma patient depends on the age of the patient, the duration of the coma, the course of the coma, and the neurologic deficits. EEG and head CT or MRI also are helpful in determining the

Table 21-1. Glasgow Coma Scale

	Score
Eye opening	
None	1
To pain	2
To verbal stimuli	3
Spontaneously	4
Best verbal response	
No response	1
Incomprehensible response	2
Inappropriate words	3
Disoriented and conversant	4
Oriented and conversant	5
Best motor response	
No response	1
Extension (decerebrate)	2
Abnormal flexion (decorticate)	3
Flexion-withdrawal to pain	4
Localizes pain	5
Obeys commands	6
Total	**15**

prognosis. Use the Glasgow Coma Scale (GCS) (Table 21-1) in determining the prognosis for postanoxic (post–cardiac arrest) or post-traumatic coma. If the patient has been paralyzed by a muscle relaxant, you cannot use this scale. Approximately 90% of patients with a GCS score of 4 or less die or remain in a PVS. Nearly 90% of patients with a GCS score of 11 or more recover or have mild to minimal disability.

22

Status Epilepticus

In this chapter, only generalized convulsive status epilepticus (SE) in adults is discussed.

WHAT YOU SHOULD KNOW

- Generalized convulsive SE is a medical emergency requiring supportive and specific therapy.
- At least 65,000 cases of SE occur each year in the United States.
- One-half of patients with SE have no history of seizures.
- SE is the initial presentation of an epileptic condition in 10% of patients.
- In approximately two-thirds of the cases of SE, there is an underlying cause or causes such as systemic metabolic derangement, drugs, hypoxia, infection, alcohol or drug withdrawal, stroke, or discontinuation of antiepileptic drugs (AEDs) (in the epileptic population).
- The longer the seizures persist, the more difficult they are to control.
- The mortality rate of SE is approximately 10% if not treated promptly.

DIAGNOSIS

Generalized convulsive SE is the state of continuous
seizures—whenever seizures persist for a sufficient length of
time (in practice, >10 minutes) or repeat frequently enough
(in practice, more than three) that full recovery of consciousness does not occur between the seizures. A **common
clinical situation** would involve a patient brought to the
emergency room because of seizures, with the duration and
number of seizures unavailable or unclear. You should wait
approximately 10 minutes before starting treatment; mean-
while, assess the patient's breathing and circulation, draw
blood for laboratory tests, and do a general physical and
neurologic examination. If the patient does not respond to
external stimuli after 10 minutes or has another seizure,
treat aggressively, because the patient is in overt SE.

Remember: It is also critical to evaluate and treat a
generalized convulsive seizure quickly if it lasts longer
than 10 minutes, because it likely represents more than a
single seizure.

MANAGEMENT

Goals of Therapy

The goals of therapy of SE are

- Stop the seizures (clinically and electrographically) as
  soon as possible (preferably within 30 minutes, but def-
  initely within 60 minutes).

- Diagnose and correct the underlying cause or causes.
- Prevent and treat systemic complications.

Guidelines for Management

In treating a patient in SE, the following guidelines are important:

- Do not panic.
- Stop seizures promptly and carefully in an organized fashion.
- Secure the airway, circulation, and cardiac status first.
- Be familiar with a treatment plan that you are comfortable with and that has been successful.
- Do not wait for results and do not change your treatment plan on the basis of AED level (persistent seizure is more harmful than a high level of AED).
- Choose an AED that can be given intravenously (IV).

Steps of Therapy

The following steps should be followed in providing therapy to a patient in SE:

1. Establish and secure the airway. Provide oxygen. If intubation becomes necessary, convulsions must be stopped first.
2. Establish two lines of IV access.
   - Open one with normal saline for IV phenytoin administration, and open one with dextrose

- Draw blood for measurement of glucose, electrolytes, complete blood cell count, toxin-drug screen, and AED levels

3. Establish a cardiac monitor and call for an electroencephalogram (EEG) if available.

4. Administer thiamine, 100 mg IV. Unless you know the patient is not hypoglycemic, administer 1 ampule (50 ml) of 50% glucose IV. A glucometer reading is not reliable, and waiting for the results of the blood sugar level test may do more harm than giving glucose empirically (some authorities do not give glucose in the early stage of SE [i.e., first 10–15 minutes] because there is release of catecholamine and secondary hyperglycemia). Hyperglycemia might cause further neuronal damage. Control blood pressure and body temperature.

5. **Terminate SE**, clinically and electrically.
   - Administer IV either lorazepam, 0.1 mg/kg at 2 mg/minute up to a total dose of 8 mg, or diazepam, 0.2 mg/kg at 5 mg/minute up to a maximum of 20 mg. Diazepam must be followed by a loading dose of phenytoin.
   - Administer phenytoin or fosphenytoin, a total dose of 20 mg/kg. Phenytoin is given at a rate of 50 mg/minute and fosphenytoin at a rate of 150 mg/minute. Watch blood pressure and heart rate. Slow down the rate if you see changes. Phenytoin is contraindicated if the patient is allergic or has an

established history of heart block. More than 80% of SE is controlled at this stage.

6. **If seizures persist, however, two options are available:**
   • Give an additional 10 mg/kg of phenytoin.
   • Consider intubation and give phenobarbital, 20 mg/kg IV at a rate of 50–100 mg/minute.

7. **If seizures persist** (refractory SE), choose one of the following options:
   • With the patient intubated and the EEG recording, initiate a pentobarbital coma. Administer a 15 mg/kg loading dose at a rate of 30 mg/minute; then give 1.5 mg/kg/hour. Continue this for 24 hours, then **try to wean** every 4–6 hours. An adequate dose of pentobarbital is judged by the appearance of burst-suppression pattern on the EEG and/or serum level of 10–20 µl/ml initially. If seizures recur while weaning, give another loading dose of pheno-barbital. Pentobarbital may cause severe hypoten-sion, requiring pressure agents (dopamine).
   • Slowly administer a loading dose of midazolam of 0.2 mg/kg and maintain at 0.75–1.00 µg/kg/minute.
   • Administer propofol, starting with 1–2 mg/kg, and maintain at 2–10 mg/kg/hour.

8. **Follow-up and maintenance**
   • If the patient presents with SE and a low level of AED, continue the same medication and improve compliance.

- If the patient had a high level of AED, consider switching to a different medication or add another AED.
- If the AED level is still low after seizures are stopped, consider a miniload (e.g., 500 mg of phenytoin orally).

KEY POINTS ABOUT STATUS EPILEPTICUS

1. The prognosis of SE depends on the duration of the seizures, promptness of treatment, adequacy of therapeutic measures, underlying cause, and age of the patient. Patients known to have epilepsy generally do well.
2. Simultaneous EEG recording is highly recommended if available:
   - To determine whether the patient is simply in a postictal state or continuing to have electrographic seizures (subclinical SE).
   - To direct therapy—for example, to determine the presence of a burst-suppression pattern when giving pentobarbital or midazolam.
   - To determine a focal abnormality, because clinically this may not be obvious in a patient with SE.
   - To determine the degree of encephalopathy.
3. Many times, the patient stops having major convulsions but remains stuporous and continues having subtle seizures such as facial muscle twitching,

twitching of the jaw and limbs, and nystagmoid eye movements. This stage is commonly known as *subtle generalized SE*, and the EEG shows periodic electrical discharges (electroclinical dissociation). This condition now is considered another end of generalized SE and is caused by a delay or inadequate therapeutic measures. It requires immediate and aggressive intervention.

4. When a patient experiences SE but his or her AED level is at a therapeutic or high level, consider an underlying metabolic or organic cause.

5. Routine administration of bicarbonate is unnecessary unless the patient is severely acidotic for a long time. Similarly, naloxone is given only when narcotic overdose is suspected.

6. Brain imaging (magnetic resonance imaging or computed tomography) should be considered in all adults with SE.

7. Lumbar puncture is indicated in febrile patients even if signs of meningitis are absent; however, lumbar puncture should be performed only when a mass lesion is excluded. Cerebrospinal fluid pleocytosis (up to 80×10^6/liter) can be seen in patients with SE.

23

Brain Edema, Transtentorial Herniation, and Increased Intracranial Pressure

BRAIN EDEMA

- Brain edema is defined as an increase in brain sodium and water content.
- It occurs in many neurologic conditions, such as stroke, trauma, tumors, infections, encephalopathies, and hydrocephalus.
- Brain edema is classified into three major types:
  - **Vasogenic:** Seen primarily in the white matter. Common causes are brain tumor, abscess, infarction, and hemorrhage. The clinical presentation is focal neurologic deficits, a decreased level of consciousness, pupillary asymmetry, and increased intracranial pressure (ICP).
  - **Cytotoxic** (cellular): Seen in the white and gray matter. Common causes are ischemic-hypoxic encephalopathies (e.g., post–cardiac arrest) and

meningitis. The clinical presentation is stupor, coma, focal or generalized seizures, and myoclonic jerks.
- **Interstitial:** Increased brain fluid due to blockage of cerebrospinal fluid absorption, seen primarily in the periventricular white matter. Common causes are pseudotumor and obstructive hydrocephalus. The clinical presentation is headache, nausea, vomiting, mental alteration, papilledema, or gait difficulty.
- Ischemic brain edema (i.e., after stroke) begins at the cellular level, then progresses to vasogenic effects. In meningitis, the edema begins at the cellular level, then changes to vasogenic, then to interstitial (resulting in hydrocephalus).

TRANSTENTORIAL HERNIATION

- Brain herniation is caused by a mass or any cause that increases ICP, thus shifting the brain substance from higher pressure to lower pressure.
- The most common cause of herniation is a transtentorial, uncal, or parahippocampal lesion.
- The clinical presentation of uncal herniation includes unilateral pupil dilation, ophthalmoplegia (due to third nerve compression), and contralateral hemiparesis, followed by ipsilateral (to the site of lesion) hemiparesis and bilateral corticospinal tract signs. These signs are followed by an irregular respiratory pattern, fixed and dilated pupils, coma, and cardiorespiratory collapse.

INCREASED INTRACRANIAL PRESSURE

- The signs of increased ICP are headache, vomiting, mental dysfunction, confusion, papilledema, decreased heart rate, decreased respiration, and increased blood pressure.
- In diagnosing patients with increased ICP, try to answer these questions:
  - Does a space-occupying lesion exist?
  - What part of the brain is involved?
  - What type of lesion is most likely the cause?
- **Remember:** A posterior fossa tumor may not have localizing signs despite signs of increased ICP.

MANAGEMENT

The following steps are taken in managing patients with brain edema, herniation, and increased ICP:

- Stabilize the patient and secure the vital signs.
- Keep the patient's head elevated.
- Keep the patient moderately dehydrated.
- Obtain a computed tomography scan or magnetic resonance imaging of the head in all patients with symptoms of increased ICP.
- **Hyperventilation:** Intubate and maintain P_{CO_2} to 25–30 mm Hg; hyperventilation immediately reduces the blood flow (vasoconstriction) and decreases ICP. Prolonged use of hyperventilation causes further ischemia to the normal and damaged brain area.

- **Hyperosmolar agents:** Mannitol is most commonly used; the dosage is 2 g/kg (25%) given in 500 ml of dextrose 5% in water (D_5W). You may repeat 0.5 g/kg every 4–6 hours. Serum osmolality is used as a treatment guide (maintain <320 mOsm/liter).
- **Diuretics:** Furosemide (Lasix) and acetazolamide (Diamox) may be helpful in pseudotumor or ischemic brain edema. The preferred dosage of furosemide is 20–40 mg intravenously (IV) every 12 hours.
- **Corticosteroids:** Dexamethasone is particularly useful in brain edema caused by primary or metastatic brain tumors or infections. The recommended loading dose is 10 mg IV, followed by 6 mg every 6 hours. The effectiveness of steroids in ischemic brain edema or cellular brain edema (hypoxia) is less clear.
- ICP monitoring is particularly useful when a patient has brain edema after head trauma.
- Eliminate or treat the underlying cause with the most effective mode of therapy. Increased ICP in many cases requires neurosurgical procedures, including hemispherectomy, ventricular drainage, and/or evacuation of a mass lesion in selected cases.

24

Metastatic Epidural Spinal Cord Compression

- Any patient diagnosed with cancer who presents with onset of persistent neck or back pain should be considered as having metastatic epidural spinal cord compression (ESCC) until proved otherwise.
- Also suspect metastatic ESCC when an elderly patient has spontaneous development of back pain.
- As many as 90% of patients with metastatic ESCC have abnormal plain spine films, showing vertebral collapse, erosion, or subluxation.
- **Magnetic resonance imaging** with contrast is the most sensitive and specific imaging technique.
- Neurologic symptoms and signs of ESCC are back and neck pain and tenderness, followed by paresthesias, sensory loss, weakness, reflex changes, and bowel and bladder dysfunction.
- In highly suspected ESCC, give a 10-mg intravenous (IV) bolus of dexamethasone followed by a 4-mg IV or oral dose every 6 hours. This treatment is followed by radiation therapy in proven cases.

- In a patient with progressive neurologic deficits, administer a 100-mg IV bolus of dexamethasone, followed by 10 mg every 6 hours. Taper off in 2–3 weeks and follow with radiation therapy.
- Surgical decompression is considered if the type of cancer is unknown, when there is neurologic deterioration after radiation, or if the tumor is resistant to radiation and there is intractable pain.

25

Acute Meningitis and Encephalitis

Acute meningitis and encephalitis are medical emergencies. If they go undiagnosed and are not treated promptly, the result is disability or death.

The clinical hallmarks of acute central nervous system (CNS) infection are fever, headaches, and nuchal rigidity, except in neonates, who may present with irritability, and the elderly, who present with changes in mental status (see Chapter 10).

ACUTE MENINGITIS

The general approach to suspected cases of acute meningitis is as follows:

- Perform a quick neurologic examination; look particularly for meningeal signs, mental status abnormalities, focal neurologic deficits, or papilledema.
- Obtain a set of blood cultures and routine admission laboratory evaluations.

- Start an intravenous (IV) line and administer broad-spectrum combination antibiotics empirically. The choice of antibiotic depends on the age of the patient.
- Administer dexamethasone, 0.15 mg/kg IV every 6 hours for 4 days to reduce complications.
- Treat seizures or electrolyte abnormalities.
- Perform a lumbar puncture (LP) as soon as possible.
- If the patient has focal neurologic signs or signs of increased intracranial pressure, obtain a computed tomography scan or magnetic resonance imaging of the head before LP.
- Record the opening pressure of cerebrospinal fluid (CSF) and send CSF for complete analysis and cultures. Save 2–3 ml of CSF for future evaluation.
- CSF analysis differentiates bacterial from viral meningitis, and the laboratory defines the antibiotic sensitivities of the infecting organism.
- The antibiotic therapy should continue for at least 10 days.
- Repeat LP approximately 48 hours after antibiotic therapy for pneumococcal meningitis.

ACUTE ENCEPHALITIS

Encephalitis is considered when the patient presents with alteration of mental state; behavioral changes or confusion; memory deficit; and focal and lateralizing neurologic signs such as paresis, aphasia, visual field defect, or focal seizures.

The leading cause of acute encephalitis is herpes simplex virus (HSV) type 1, which affects the frontotemporal lobe unilaterally or bilaterally. HSV encephalitis is a medical emergency and should be considered in a patient who presents with encephalitic features until proved otherwise.

The general approach to **suspected cases of acute encephalitis** is as follows:

- Begin IV antiviral therapy with acyclovir, 10 mg/kg every 8 hours for 14 days, and monitor kidney function.
- Perform an LP; the CSF composition in HSV encephalitis is similar to that of any viral meningitis except it has a higher concentration of protein and higher rate of xanthochromia.
- The most specific and sensitive test for HSV encephalitis is measurement of the virus DNA by polymerase chain reaction, which is very useful in the early stage of the disease.
- Head imaging such as computed tomography scan or magnetic resonance imaging may identify an abnormal signal in the temporal lobe. The typical electroencephalographic feature is occurrence of periodic or quasiperiodic lateralized epileptiform discharges over the temporal lobe.
- Brain biopsy may be considered when the neurologic status deteriorates despite acyclovir therapy.

RULE OF THUMB

In suspected cases of acute bacterial meningitis, initiate IV combination antibiotic therapy and perform an LP as soon as possible. In suspected cases of encephalitis, initiate IV acyclovir.

26

Delirium Tremens

WHAT YOU SHOULD KNOW

- Delirium tremens (DTs) is a medical emergency.
- It occurs in approximately 30% of patients who present with alcohol withdrawal seizures.
- The onset of DTs is acute, manifesting as profound confusion, delusion, vivid visual hallucinations, tremor, agitation, insomnia, nausea and vomiting, and autonomic hyperactivity (dilated pupils, fever, tachycardia, profuse sweating, orthostatic hypotension).
- The onset of DTs is 72–96 hours after cessation of alcohol intake (patients are often hospitalized for a different reason) and usually resolves 3–4 days after treatment.
- Patients with DTs should be investigated for underlying medical conditions such as infection, pancreatitis, liver disease, or subdural hematoma.
- Mortality from DTs in untreated cases is approximately 15%, due to circulatory collapse, hyperthermia, or infection.

- Although the diagnosis of DTs is clinical, all patients should have these tests: complete blood cell count, coagulation studies, serum amylase, blood chemistry, chest x-ray, lumbar puncture, and head computed tomography scan.
- Although DTs is not due to thiamine deficiency, thiamine is given to prevent the development of Wernicke's encephalopathy.

MANAGEMENT

The following steps are taken in the management of DTs:

- Stabilize and monitor vital signs.
- Hydrate the patient well (sometimes 6–8 liters/day is needed); use more normal saline fluid.
- Add B-complex vitamins to each fluid bag.
- Restrain the patient if necessary to prevent injury.
- Calm the patient with short-acting sedatives such as diazepam or lorazepam. Diazepam is given 10 mg intravenously (IV) followed by 5 mg every 10 minutes until the patient is calm, and maintain with 5 mg every 1–4 hours as necessary.
- Administer thiamine, 200 mg IV, then 100 mg per day for several days.
- Correct any electrolyte abnormalities (hypomagnesemia, hypokalemia, hypocalcemia, or hypoglycemia).
- Treat coexistent medical conditions such as infection and pancreatitis. Reduce hyperthermia with a cooling blanket.

- Beta-adrenergic blockers (e.g., atenolol) or alpha$_2$-adrenergic agents (e.g., clonidine) may be used to reduce autonomic hyperactivities.

A COMMON MISTAKE

Oversedation of patients with DTs is not only misleading clinically (supressing mental alertness), it depresses cardiopulmonary function.

27

Wernicke's Encephalopathy

WHAT YOU SHOULD KNOW

- Wernicke's encephalopathy (WE) is caused by a thiamine deficiency and is seen commonly in chronic alcoholics. It is also seen in patients in any poor nutritional state (e.g., due to hypoalimentation, cancer, starvation, chronic gastrointestinal disease, acquired immunodeficiency syndrome).
- The onset of WE is acute or subacute. Typical clinical features include
  - **Global confusional state: apathy, disorientation, confusion, lethargy.** Rarely, stupor and coma are reported. Remember that 5–10% of patients with WE may have normal mental status.
  - **Eye abnormalities:** nystagmus (horizontal or vertical), lateral rectus weakness (diplopia), gaze palsy, total external ophthalmoplegia, and, rarely, ptosis and retinal changes.
  - **Ataxia** (truncal): difficulty in stance and gait.
- Isolated signs (e.g., ophthalmoplegia alone) in an alcoholic do not exclude the diagnosis.

- Most patients with WE have signs and symptoms of peripheral neuropathy.
- The diagnosis of WE is primarily clinical, but an abnormality in cold caloric testing and reduced red blood cell transketolase are seen.
- Response to therapy (thiamine) is good and often complete in cases of ophthalmoplegia, but recovery from ataxia and mental confusion may be slow and incomplete.
- Untreated WE leads to Korsakoff's psychosis and has a 10% chance of fatality.

MANAGEMENT

The following steps are taken in the management of WE:

- Hospitalize the patient.
- Administer thiamine parenterally (200-mg loading dose) followed by 100 mg every day for 3–4 days; continue with 100 mg orally twice a day with vitamin B complex.
- Improve the nutritional state of the patient.
- Search for and treat the underlying medical condition (infection, pancreatitis, electrolyte abnormalities).

COMMON MISTAKES

- Use of a high-carbohydrate diet or high-glucose solution without adding adequate supplemental thiamine causes further depletion of thiamine reserves.
- Rapid correction of hyponatremia may lead to quadriplegia (central pontine myelinolysis).

28

Myasthenia Gravis Crisis

WHAT YOU SHOULD KNOW

- Crisis in myasthenia gravis (MG) is defined as rapidly progressively respiratory and bulbar muscle weakness.
- In evaluating a patient in crisis, do not spend too much time trying to determine whether the crisis is **myasthenic** or **cholinergic**. This differentiation is not only unnecessary but also often difficult. **Your main goal is to keep the patient alive.**
- The mortality rate from crisis is now approximately 5%, compared with 50% three decades ago.
- It is important to recognize and treat **impending crisis**; impending crisis is suspected when the patient has sleeping difficulties, tachycardia, dyspnea, and dysphagia.
- The goal of therapy is to strengthen respiratory and bulbar muscles; less important are the limb and eye muscles.
- Try to identify underlying causes for crisis, such as infection, electrolyte abnormalities, stress, and excessive use of cholinesterase inhibitors. In many cases, the cause of crisis remains unknown.

- **Remember:** When a patient is in crisis, treat the infection aggressively with the best available antibiotic. Do not be concerned that the antibiotic may adversely affect neuromuscular transmission.
- During an MG crisis, it is best and most practical to stop all cholinesterase inhibitors for these reasons:
  - The patient is now in the intensive care unit and resting.
  - These drugs cause excessive tracheal secretions, their effect is transient, and they may worsen "cholinergic" crisis.
- It is good practice to transfer stable patients to the nearest medical center equipped with a plasma exchange facility.

MANAGEMENT

The following steps are taken in the management of patients in MG crisis:

- Secure the airway and stabilize the patient.
- Obtain chest x-ray, forced vital capacity, and arterial blood gases.
- Electively intubate the patient when forced vital capacity is less than 12 ml/kg.
- Stop all cholinesterase inhibitors (e.g., pyridostigmine [Mestinon]).
- Admit the patient to the intensive care unit.
- Arrange for plasma exchange (see Chapter 19).

- Identify and treat the underlying cause aggressively.
- If plasma exchange is not available, you may consider use of intravenous immunoglobulin (see Chapter 19), although its effectiveness in crisis is less clear, or increase the dosage of corticosteroid (e.g., methylprednisolone [Solu-Medrol]).
- Cholinesterase inhibitors may be reinstituted after 48–72 hours, with a lower dose and gradual titration.

A COMMON MISTAKE

You receive a call from your patient stating the cholinesterase inhibitor (**Mestinon**) is **no longer** helpful and he or she is having difficulty sleeping and swallowing. Do not adjust or increase the Mestinon dosage by telephone. Assess the patient in your office or the emergency room for impending crisis.

29

Guillain-Barré Syndrome

WHAT YOU SHOULD KNOW

- Guillain-Barré syndrome (GBS) is the most common cause of acute, generalized motor paralysis in developed countries.
- It is also the most common cause of acute demyelinating polyneuropathy caused by immune attack (cellular and humoral factors) against the myelin sheath.
- Weakness starts in the legs, with proximal distribution and minimal sensory loss.
- Any patient who presents acutely with symmetric, proximal weakness associated with decreased or absent muscle stretch reflexes should be considered as having GBS until proved otherwise.
- The weakness evolves within days to weeks, most commonly peaking in 2–3 weeks.
- Cranial nerve and respiratory muscle weakness usually occurs later.
- Doubt the diagnosis of GBS if the patient has preserved reflexes despite significant weakness, has persistent segmental or unilateral sensory loss, has developed

bowel and bladder dysfunction initially, or atypical electrophysiologic features and persistently high elevated cerebrospinal fluid (CSF) cell count.

- The most important diagnostic tests are CSF examination, which typically shows high elevation of protein concentration but no rise or minimal rise of cell count (*albumino-cytologic dissociation*), and nerve conduction studies (NCSs) and needle electromyography (EMG), which show demyelinating neuropathy. Remember, however, that NCSs and EMG may not show changes for the first week. In the early stages of the disease, F waves, however, may be prolonged or absent. Reduced amplitude of motor response generally implies a poor prognosis.

- The prognosis of GBS is good, with complete recovery in as many as 80% of patients; significant disability in approximately 15%; and mortality in approximately 5% due to dysautonomia, cardiac arrest, sepsis, pulmonary embolism, or acute respiratory distress syndrome. Recurrence rates are 2–5% after complete recovery and 10% before complete recovery.

- Intravenous immunoglobulin is shown to be as effective and readily available as plasma exchange in the treatment of GBS. It is also safer.

MANAGEMENT

The following steps are taken in the management of patients with GBS:

- Admit the patient to the intensive care unit.
- Assure the patient about a good chance of recovery with effective therapy despite progressive worsening.
- Monitor respiratory function; if forced vital capacity is less than 12–15 ml/kg, consider elective intubation.
- **Bedside hint:** If the patient can count to 25 in one breath, the forced vital capacity is approximately 2 liters; if the patient can count to 10, it is 1 liter.
- Arrange for plasmapheresis if the patient is rapidly worsening. Remove 200–250 ml/kg of plasma in four to six exchanges on alternate days and replace with 5% albumin. Rare complications of exchange include hypotension, bleeding tendency, and cardiac arrhythmia. Hepatitis and acquired immunodeficiency syndrome are risks if plasma is used as a replacement.
- If plasmapheresis is unavailable or the patient is unstable, intravenous immunoglobulin is as effective as plasmapheresis. The dosage is 400 mg/kg for 5 consecutive days.
- Further subacute and long-term therapeutic measures are nursing, management of autonomic dysfunction, prevention of infection, controlling bladder function, deep venous thrombosis and pulmonary embolism prophylaxis, and physical therapy.

Temporal Arteritis

WHAT YOU SHOULD KNOW

- Temporal arteritis (TA) is a medical emergency; if undiagnosed and untreated, it causes permanent blindness or even stroke.
- In an elderly individual with new onset of severe, unilateral or bilateral, persistent headache or head pain, TA should be considered until proved otherwise.
- The typical presentation of TA is unilateral or bilateral boring headaches, head pain, or scalp tenderness (felt when brushing hair or wearing a hat). The temporal artery is usually tender, nodular, and unpulsatile. Constitutional symptoms include anorexia, weight loss, malaise, generalized myalgia (polymyalgia rheumatica), and visual symptoms.
- Vision loss, once present, is usually permanent.
- The most important diagnostic tests are markedly elevated erythrocyte sedimentation rate (ESR) (at least greater than the patient's age) and C-reactive protein (CRP).
- Definitive diagnosis is made by temporal artery biopsy (TAB), demonstrating granulomatous inflammation.

- Normal ESR occurs in approximately 10% of biopsy-proven cases. A normal TAB may be seen because of a "skip lesion." Onset before age 40 and the absence of headaches are very rare.
- TAB should not be considered negative unless both temporal arteries are biopsied and an adequate length (5 cm) is taken.

MANAGEMENT

The following steps are taken in the management of TA:

- In suspected cases of TA, order ESR and CRP. ESR should be measured as soon as blood is drawn; a delay in measurement may falsely show a low level.
- Begin corticosteroid (prednisone), 60–80 mg per day orally, and schedule the patient for TAB (of the more symptomatic side).
- Do not delay therapy by waiting for biopsy results because prednisone does not effect histologic changes for up to 72 hours.
- Patients who present with visual symptoms should be treated initially with intravenous steroid (e.g., methyl-prednisolone, 250 mg qid for 3–5 days) followed by a high dose of oral prednisone (e.g., 80 mg/day).
- High-dose oral prednisone should be continued until ESR is normalized (2–3 months), then tapered slowly to the lowest effective dose (6–12 months). Most

patients require prednisone therapy for 1–2 years.
Alternate-day prednisone is not as effective. Monitor
ESR, visual symptoms, and steroid complications.
- When vision loss has occurred in one eye, you should
be aggressive with therapy to protect the other eye.

Index

Acetylcholinesterase inhibitors, for treatment of
      myasthenia gravis, 265, 266
Acquired immunodeficiency syndrome. *See* AIDS
Acute disseminated encephalomyelitis, 172–173
Acute transverse myelitis. *See* Transverse myelitis, acute
Acyclovir, in acute encephalitis, 319
Adie's pupil, 13
Adrenergic tests, 101
Agnosia, testing for, 7–8
Agraphesthesia, 8
AIDS, 150–152
   encephalopathy, 152
   myelopathy, 152
   neurologic complications of, 150–152
Alcohol
   neurologic complications of, 179–182
      cerebellar degeneration, 182
      nutritional polyneuropathy, 181–182
      withdrawal seizures, 180–181
   for treatment of essential tremor, 230
Alpha waves, in electroencephalography, 95
Alteration of mental status, 153–162. *See also* Delirium; Dementia
   electroencephalography in, 97
Alzheimer's disease, 157–158
   cognition in, 158
   depression in, 158
   diagnosis of, 157
   disease progression in, 158
   sleep disorders in, 158
   treatment of, 157
Amantadine hydrochloride, in therapy for Parkinson's disease, 228

Amitriptyline
    in prophylaxis of migraine, 198
    in treatment of trigeminal neuralgia, 208
Amyotrophic lateral sclerosis, 252–254
    diagnosis of, 243
    therapy for, 254
Anatomy. *See* Neuroanatomy
Angiography
    cerebral, 84–85
    magnetic resonance, 85
Anisocoria, 13
Anosmia, 10–11
Anterior horn cells, 247
    lesions affecting, 73–74
Anticholinergics
    for symptoms of dizziness, 188
    in therapy for Parkinson's disease, 228
Anticoagulant therapy, for stroke prevention, 120, 131–132
Antiepileptic drugs, 138
    in alcohol withdrawal seizures, 181
    new, 142–143
    in pregnancy, 139–140
    in prophylaxis of migraine, 198
    withdrawal of, 141–142
Antihistamines
    in prophylaxis of migraine, 198
    for symptoms of dizziness, 188
Antiplatelet therapy, for stroke prevention, 120
Aphasia, 132–133
Apneustic respiratory pattern, in coma, 300
Apraxia, testing for, 7–8
Argyll-Robertson pupils, 14
Arsenic poisoning, 222
Arterial dissection, 127–128
Astereognosis, 8
Ataxic respiratory pattern, in coma, 300
Atenolol, in prophylaxis of migraine, 198
Athetosis, definition of, 224

Autonomic function tests, 100–102
Azathioprine, in treatment of myasthenia gravis, 267–268

Babinski's sign, 41, 42
Back and neck pain, 283–288
    diagnostic tests for, 287
    evaluation of, 285–287
        focused neurologic examination, 286–287
        history, 285–286
        physical examination, 286
    treatment of, 288
Baclofen, in treatment of trigeminal neuralgia, 208
Ballismus, definition of, 224
Barber's chair sign, 53
Bell's palsy, 216, 255–256
Benign paroxysmal positional vertigo, 186
Benzodiazepines, for symptoms of dizziness, 188
Benztropine mesylate, in therapy of Parkinson's disease, 228
Beta blockers, in prophylaxis of migraine, 198
Beta waves, in electroencephalography, 95
Biopsies, 106–108
    brain, 106–107
    leptomeningeal, 107
    muscle, 107–108
    nerve, 108
    temporal artery, 107
Bitemporal hemianopia, 15
Blood tests
    in back and neck pain, 287
    for diagnosis of neuromuscular diseases, 249
Borderzone infarcts, 68
Botulism, 272
Brachial plexitis, nontraumatic adult-onset, 250–251
Bradykinesia, in Parkinson's disease, 225–226
Brain biopsy, 106–107
Brain death, 293
Brain edema. *See* Edema, brain
Brain stem auditory evoked potentials, 93–94

Brain stem lesion
   extra-axial, 70
   hallmarks of, 70
Brandt-Daroff exercise, 188
Bromocriptine, in therapy for Parkinson's disease, 229
Brown-Séquard syndrome, 71–72
Brudzinski's sign, 54
Bruxism, 241

Calcium channel blockers, in prophylaxis of migraine, 198
Caloric test, 26, 299
Carbamazepine, in treatment of trigeminal neuralgia, 208
Cardiovagal heart rate response test, 101
Carotid dissection, 128
Carotid Doppler ultrasonography, 85
Carotid endarterectomy, for stroke prevention, 120
Carpal tunnel syndrome, 54, 217, 256–257
Catechol methyltransferase inhibitors, in therapy for
        Parkinson's disease, 229
Cauda equina syndrome, 72
Cavernous sinus thrombosis, eye symptoms in, 206
Central nervous system infections, 145–152. *See also* AIDS; Meningitis;
      Neurosyphilis
   Creutzfeldt-Jakob disease, 150
   diagnostic studies in, 145
   symptoms of, 145
   therapy for, 145
Central nervous system vasculitis, 128–129
Central pontine myelinolysis, 176–177
Central sleep apnea syndrome, 239
Cerebellar function. *See* Coordination
Cerebellar lesions, 73
Cerebral aneurysm. *See* Subarachnoid hemorrhage
Cerebral angiography, 84–85
Charcot-Marie-Tooth disease, 214, 221, 260–261
Cheyne-Stokes pattern, 300
Cholinesterase inhibitors, in myasthenia gravis crisis, 330–331
Chorea, definition of, 224
Circumduction, 45

Clonazepam
    for restless legs syndrome, 242
    for sleep myoclonus, 242
    in treatment of trigeminal neuralgia, 208
Clostridium botulinum, 272
Clumsy hand syndrome, 71
Cluster headache, 199–200
Cocaine test, 109–110
Cogwheel rigidity, in Parkinson's disease, 225
Coma, 293–303
    as medical emergency, 294
    differential diagnosis in, 301–302
    electroencephalography in, 97–98
    history and physical examination in, 295
    laboratory studies, 302
    neurologic examination in, 296–301
        abnormal postures, 300
        appearance of patient, 296
        eyes, 296
            movements of, 298–299
            pupils, 297
        head and neck, 296
        motor response, 299–300
        other neurologic signs, 301
        respiratory pattern, 300–301
    prognosis in, 302–303
    stabilization of patient in, 294–295
    terminology, 293
Computed tomography, 81–82
    in diagnosis of dementia, 162
Conductive hearing loss, 25
Conjugate eye deviation, 298
Conus medullaris syndrome, 72
Coordination, 45–49
    lower extremity, 47
        foot or heel tapping testing for, 47
        heel-to-shin testing for, 47
        heel-to-toe testing for, 47
    trunk, 47–48

Coordination (*continued*)
   upper extremity, 45–47
      alternate rebound test for, 47
      finger-to-nose test for, 46
      rapid alternating movements test for, 46
      rebound test for, 46
Copolymer-1 (Copaxone), in multiple sclerosis, 170
Corticobulbar tract, 64
Corticospinal tract, 64
Corticosteroids
   for carpal tunnel syndrome, 257
   in management of brain edema, herniation, and increased intracranial
         pressure, 314
   for prophylaxis of cluster headache, 200
   in treatment of myasthenia gravis, 267
Cranial nerve dysfunction, sources of, 9–10.
Cranial nerve (CN) examination, 9–30
   anatomy, 9
   CN I (olfactory), 10–11
   CNs II, III, IV, VI (eye), 11–20. *See also* Eye, examination of
   CNs V and VII (face), 20–24. *See also* Facial nerve, examination of;
         Trigeminal nerve, examination of
   CN VIII (hearing and vestibular), 24–26. *See also* Hearing, examina-
         tion of; Vestibular system, examination of
   CNs IX, X, XII (mouth), 27–29. *See also* Mouth, examination of
   CN XI (shoulders and neck), 29–30
Cranial nerve palsy, 19
Creutzfeldt-Jakob disease, 150
   electroencephalography in, 98
Cubital tunnel syndrome, 217, 257–258
Cyproheptadine, in prophylaxis of migraine, 198

Dejerine-Sottas, 260–261
Delirium, 153–155
   causes of, 154–155
   hallmarks of, 153–154
Delirium tremens, 321–323
   management of, 322–323
   oversedation of patients with, 323

Delta waves, in electroencephalography, 95
Dementia, 8–9, 156–162
    causes of, 157–159
        Alzheimer's disease, 157–158. *See also* Alzheimer's disease
        dementia with Lewy bodies, 159
        vascular or multi-infarct dementia, 159
    differential diagnosis of, 156
    evaluation of patient with, 160–161
    incidence of, 156
    parkinsonian features and, 159
    workup for, 161–162
Demyelinating disorders, 163–177. *See also* Isolated idiopathic optic
                neuritis; Multiple sclerosis; Transverse myelitis, acute
    acute disseminated encephalomyelitis, 172–173
    central pontine myelinolysis, 176–177
    progressive multifocal leukoencephalopathy, 176
Dermatomes, 65
Dexamethasone
    in management of brain edema, herniation, and increased intracranial
                pressure, 314
    in treatment of status migrainosus, 199
    in treatment of acute meningitis, 318
Diabetic amyotrophy, 259
Diabetic neuropathies, 259
Diagnostic tests and procedures, 79–110. *See also* Biopsies; Electrophys-
                iologic tests; Lumbar puncture; Neuroimaging; Pharmaco-
                logic tests
    ischemic exercise forearm test, 108–109
3',4'-Diaminopyrimidine, in treatment of Lambert-Eaton myasthenic
                syndrome, 271
Diazepam, in delirium tremens, 322
Dihydroergotamine, for treatment of migraine,
                196, 199
Dimenhydrinate, for symptoms of dizziness, 188
Diplopia, 18
Directional scratch test, 34
Disconjugate gaze palsy, 19
Dissection, arterial, 127–128
Disseminated encephalomyelitis, acute, 172–173

Diuretics
  in management of brain edema, herniation, and increased intracranial
        pressure, 314
  for symptoms of dizziness, 188
Divalproex
  in prophylaxis of migraine, 198
  in treatment of trigeminal neuralgia, 208
Dizziness
  drug-induced, 185–186
  evaluation of patient with, 187
  key points in history of patient with, 183
  key points in physical examination of patient with, 184
  symptomatic drug therapy for, 188
"Doll's eye" test, 298–299
Dopamine agonists, in therapy for Parkinson's disease, 228–229
Dorsal column (lemniscal) tract, 64
Double simultaneous stimulation, 35
Doxepin, in prophylaxis of migraine, 198
Drug-induced extrapyramidal syndromes. *See* Extrapyramidal syn-
        dromes, drug-induced
Dysdiadochokinesia, 46
Dysmetria, 46
Dystonia, 38
  acute drug-induced, 232
  definition of, 224

Edema, brain, 311–314
  cytotoxic, 311–312
  interstitial, 312
  ischemic, 312
  management of, 313–314
  vasogenic, 311
Edrophonium test, 109
  for myasthenia gravis, 262–263
Electroencephalography, 95–99
  in acute encephalitis, 319
  in alcohol withdrawal seizures, 181
  in alteration of mental state, 97

in brain death, 99
in coma, electroencephalography in, 97–98
in epilepsy, 96–97, 136
    in surgery for, 98
in infection, 98
and non–rapid eye movement sleep, 235
in pseudoepilepsy, 98
in status epilepticus, 97
wave forms in, 95–96
Electromyography
    in back and neck pain, 287
    in myotonic muscular dystrophy, 279
    needle, 88, 90–91
    single-fiber, 92
        in myasthenia gravis, 263–264
Electrophysiologic tests, 88–102
    autonomic function tests, 100–102
    electroencephalography, 95–99. *See also* Electroencephalography
    evoked potentials, 92–95. *See also* Evoked potentials
    in Lambert-Eaton myasthenic syndrome, 271
    needle electromyography, 88, 90–91
    in neuromuscular diseases, 249
        in myasthenia gravis, 263–264
    nerve conduction studies, 88–89
    in peripheral neuropathy, 213
    repetitive nerve stimulation, 91–92
    single-fiber electromyography, 92
    sleep studies, 99–100
Embolic stroke, 123–124
Encephalitis, acute, 318–320
Enuresis, 240–241
Epicritic pain, therapy for, 221
Epilepsy. *See also* Seizures
    definition of, 135
    and driving, 140
    in elderly, 140–141
    electroencephalography in, 96–97
    surgery for, 98

Ergotamine, for treatment of migraine, 195–196
Essential tremor, 229–231
    clinical features of, 229–230
    treatment, 230–231
Evoked potentials, 92–95
    brain stem auditory evoked, 93–94
    in diagnosis of multiple sclerosis, 167–168
    somatosensory evoked, 94–95
    visual evoked, 93
Excessive daytime sleepiness (narcolepsy), 238–239
Extrapyramidal syndromes, drug-induced, 231–233
    acute drug-induced dystonia, 232
    tardive dyskinesia, 232–233
Eye, examination of, 11–20
    fundi, 15–16
    movement, 16–20
        abnormalities of, 17–18, 19–20
        in coma, 298–299
        nystagmus, 18–19
    ptosis, 12
    pupils, 12–14. *See also* Pupils
    visual acuity, 14
    visual field, 14–15

Fabry's disease, 212, 222
Facial nerve, examination of, 22–24
    asymmetry, 23
    lower motor neuron weakness, 23–24, 73
    upper motor neuron weakness, 24, 73
Facial pain, 207–208. *See also* Trigeminal neuralgia
Fasciculation, 38–39, 90
Fascioscapulohumeral muscular dystrophy, 279–280
Felbamate, 142
Fibrillation potentials, 90
Finger tapping test, 39
Fisher's sign, 57
Foot circling sign, 39
Footdrop, 45, 76–77, 258–259
Forearm rolling test, 39, 57

Formulation, neurologic, 51–52
Froment's paper sign, 54
Fundoscopy, 15–16
Furosemide, in management of brain edema, herniation, and increased
            intracranial pressure, 314

Gabapentin, 142
    in treatment of trigeminal neuralgia, 208
Gag reflex, testing of, 28
Gait, 44
    abnormal, 44–45
        antalgic, 45
        apraxia, 44
        ataxia, 44
        circumduction, 45
        footdrop, 45
        functional, 45
        marche à petits pas, 45
        scissoring, 45
        steppage, 45
        waddling, 45
    examination of, 44
Gegenhalten, 38
Gerstmann's syndrome, 8, 67–68
Glabellar reflex, 43
Glasgow Coma Scale, 303
Gottren's papules, in dermatomyositis, 274
Grasp reflex, 43
Guillain-Barré syndrome, 333–335
    diagnostic tests for, 334
    management of, 335
    prognosis in, 334

Hallpike's test, 56
Hand-muscle weakness and atrophy, 75
Head-tilt test, 56
Headache, 189–207
    analgesic-rebound, 201
    caused by pseudotumor cerebri. *See* Pseudotumor cerebri

Headache (*continued*)
  chronic daily, 201
  cluster, 199–200
  diagnostic tests for, 204–206
    in acute meningitis, 206
    in basilar-artery migraine, 205
    in "first or worst headache in life," 205
    in pseudotumor cerebri, 204–205
    in temporal arteritis, 205
    in spontaneous internal carotid artery dissection, 206
    in "thunderclap headache," 205
  evaluation of, 189–190
    history, 189
    laboratory tests, 190
    physical and neurologic examination, 190
  hospitalization for, 204
  migraine, 193–199. *See also* Migraine
  ophthalmology and, 206–207
  post-traumatic, 202
  tension-type, 191
Hearing, examination of, 24–25
Hearing loss, conductive vs. sensorineural, 25
Herpes simplex encephalitis, electroencephalography in, 98
Higher cortical function, testing of, 6–9. *See also* Mental status,
      testing of
History, neurologic, 5–6
Hoffmann's reflex, 43
Homonymous hemianopia, 15
Homonymous quadrantanopia, 15
Hoover's sign, 55–56
Horner's syndrome, 13
Hydrochlorothiazide, for symptoms of dizziness, 188
Hyperosmolar agents, in management of brain edema, herniation, and
      increased intracranial pressure, 314
Hyperventilation
  in coma, 301
  in management of brain edema, herniation, and increased intracranial
      pressure, 313

Hyposmia, 10–11
Hypoventilation, in coma, 301

Immunoglobulin, intravenous
    in Guillain-Barré syndrome, 334
    in treatment of myasthenia gravis, 268
Immunosuppressive drugs, in treatment of myasthenia gravis, 267–268
Infections. *See* Central nervous system infections
Insomnias, 237
Interferon B-Ia (Avonex), in multiple sclerosis, 170
Interferon B-Ib (Betaseron), in multiple sclerosis, 170
Internuclear ophthalmoplegia, 17, 19, 68
    bilateral, 19–20
Intracerebral hemorrhage, spontaneous, 124–125
Intracranial pressure, increased, 312
    management of, 313–314
Intrathecal therapy, 104
Ischemic exercise forearm test, 108–109
Isolated idiopathic optic neuritis, 173–174
    clinical features of, 173
    examination for, 173–174
    and multiple sclerosis, 174
    therapy for, 174
Isometheptene, for treatment of migraine, 197
Jannetta procedure, 208
Jaw jerk reflex, 43
Joint position sense, testing for, 33–34
Jolly test, in myasthenia gravis, 263

Kernig's sign, 54

Labetalol, in hypertensive stroke patient, 116
Labyrinthitis, acute, 186–187
Lacunar stroke, 122–123
Lambert-Eaton myasthenic syndrome, 270–271
    clinical features of, 270
    diagnostic tests for, 270–271
    treatment of, 271

Lamotrigine, 142
Lateral gaze palsy, 19
Lateral medullary syndrome, 69
Leptomeningeal biopsy, 107
Levodopa, in therapy of Parkinson's disease, 228
Lewy bodies, dementia with, 159
Lhermitte's sign, 53
Lithium carbonate, for prophylaxis of cluster headache, 200
Locked-in syndrome, 293
Low back pain, in elderly, 284
Lower motor neuron weakness, 23–24
Lumbar puncture, 103–106
    contraindications for, 105–106
    complications of, 106
    in diagnosis of dementia, 162
    indications for
        anesthetic, 104
        diagnostic, 103
        therapeutic, 104
    precautions in suspected bloody tap, 105
    procedure for, 104–105
Lumbar stenosis, 285

Macular sparing, 15
Magnetic resonance angiography, 85
Magnetic resonance imaging, 82–83
Marchiafava-Bignami syndrome, 179
Marcus Gunn pupil, 13, 53
Meclizine hydrochloride, for symptoms of dizziness, 188
Medial longitudinal fasciculus, 65
Meningitis, 146–148
    acute, approach to suspected cases of, 317–318, 320
    bacterial, 146–147
        complications of, 147
        leading pathogens in, 146
        recurrent, 147
        risk factors for, 146–147
    tuberculous, 148
    viral (aseptic), 147–148

Mental status, testing of, 6–9
    Mini-Mental State Examination for. *See* Mini-Mental State Examination
Meralgia paresthetica, 218
Metabolic myopathies, 280–281
Methylprednisolone
    for acute disseminated encephalomyelitis, 173
    for acute exacerbations of multiple sclerosis, 169
Methysergide, in prophylaxis of migraine, 198
Meyerson's reflex, 43
Migraine
    aura without headache, 194
    basilar-artery, 194
        diagnostic tests in, 205
    complicated, 193
    during pregnancy, 201–202
    eye symptoms in, 206
    infarction, 193
        diagnostic tests in, 205
    transformed, 201
    treatment of, 194–199
        nonpharmacologic, 194–195
        pharmacologic, 195–198
            abortive symptomatic, 195
                dihydroergotamine, 196
                ergotamines, 195–196
                serotonin receptor agonists, 196–197
            nonspecific symptomatic, 195
            prophylactic, 197–198
            for status migrainosus, 198–199
    with aura, 192–193
    without aura, 193
Mini-Mental State Examination, 7–8
    interpretation of, 8
        in evaluating patient with dementia, 160
Mononeuropathy multiplex, 217, 219
Motor nerve conduction studies, 89
Motor neuron disease, 250, 252–254. *See also* Amyotrophic
                lateral sclerosis
    clinical characteristics of, 250

Motor system examination, 36–49
  approach in, for patient with suspected dysfunction, 44
  coordination and cerebellar function, 45–49. *See also* Coordination
  gait, 44–45. *See also* Gait
  reflexes, 40–43. *See also* Reflexes
  muscle atrophy and fasciculation, 38–39
  muscle tone, 37–38
Motor unit, 247
Mouth, examination of, 27–29
  larynx, 28–29
  pharynx, 28
  tongue, 27–28
Movement disorders, 223–233. *See also* Essential tremor;
        Parkinson's disease
  evaluation for, 223
  drug-induced, 231–233. *See also* Extrapyramidal syndromes,
        drug-induced
  myoclonus, 233
  terminology for abnormal movements, 223–225
Multiple sclerosis, 163–171
  and acute transverse myelitis, 175
  clinical course of, 164
  diagnosis of, 165–168
    cerebrospinal fluid abnormalities and, 167
    evoked potentials and, 167–168
    history and examination for, 165–166
    magnetic resonance imaging of brain for, 166–167
  initial presentation of, 164
  and isolated idiopathic optic neuritis, 174
  prognosis in, 168
  symptoms and signs suggestive of, 164–165
  therapy for, 169–171
    in acute exacerbations, 169
    rehabilitative, 171
    in relapsing remitting cases, 169–170
    for symptoms, 170–171
Multiple sleep latency test, 100
Muscle atrophy, 38

Muscle biopsy, 107–108
Muscle disease, primary. *See* Myopathy
Muscle fibers, 247–248
Muscle sprain, 283
Muscle tone, examination of, 37–38
Muscle weakness, 36–37
Muscular dystrophy, 277–280
    cause of, 277
    diagnosis of, 277
    fascioscapulohumeral, 279–280
    myotonic, 278–279
Myasthenia gravis, 261–269
    cause of, 261
    clinical hallmarks of, 262
    clinical pearls, 268–269
    crisis, 329–331
        management of, 330–331
        stopping cholinesterase inhibitors in, 330
    diagnosis of, 262–265
        acetylcholine receptor antibody test, 264
        autoantibodies, 264
        blood tests, 264–265
        edrophonium (Tensilon) test, 262–263
        electrophysiologic tests, 263–264
        imaging, 265
    single-fiber electromyography in, 92, 263–264
    treatment of, 265–268
        guidelines for, 266–268
        immunosuppressive, 265, 267–268
        symptomatic, 265
        thymectomy, 267–268, 269
Myelography, 84
Myoclonus, definition of, 224
Myopathy, 77, 273–281. *See also* Muscular dystrophy
    clinical characteristics of, 252
    congenital, 276–277
    dermatomyositis, 274–275
    inclusion body myositis, 275–276

Myopathy (*continued*)
  polymyositis, 273–274
  metabolic, 280–281
Myotonia, 38
Myotonic muscular dystrophy, 278–279

Naproxen, in prophylaxis of migraine, 198
Naratriptan, for treatment of migraine, 197
Narcolepsy, 238–239
Neck, examination of, 29–30
Neck pain. *See* Back and neck pain
Needle electromyography, 88, 90–91
Nerve biopsy, 108
Nerve conduction studies, 88–89
  in back and neck pain, 287
Neuroanatomy, 63–65
  corticobulbar tract, 64
  corticospinal tract, 64
  dermatomes, 65
  dorsal column (lemniscal) tract, 64
  medial longitudinal fasciculus, 65
  spinothalamic tract, 64
  visual tract (straight), 65
Neuroimaging, 81–88
  in back and neck pain, 287
  carotid Doppler ultrasonography, 85
  cerebral angiography, 84–85
  computed tomography, 81–82
  magnetic resonance angiography, 85
  magnetic resonance imaging, 82–83
  myelography, 84
  in neuromuscular diseases, 249
  positron emission tomography, 86–87
  single-photon emission computed tomography, 87–88
  transcranial Doppler ultrasonography, 86
  x-rays, 81
Neuroleptics, as cause of extrapyramidal syndromes, 231–232

Neurologic examination, 3–49
cranial nerve examination, 9–30. *See also* Cranial nerve (CN)
examination
length of, 4
mental status and higher cortical function examination, 6–9. *See also*
Mental status, testing of
modified, 51–52
motor system examination, 36–49. *See also* Motor system examination
purpose of, 4
sensory, 30–35. *See also* Sensory examination
sequence of, 4
taking a history, 5–6
Neurologic history, 5–6
Neuromuscular diseases, 247–281. *See also* Motor neuron disease;
Myopathy; Neuromuscular junction disorders; Presynaptic
disorders
anatomy, 247–248
diagnosis of, 249–252
diagnostic tests for, 249
evaluation of patient with, 248–249
nontraumatic adult-onset brachial plexitis, 250–251
polyneuropathies, 251. *See also* Peripheral neuropathy
signs of, 248–249
symptoms of, 248
Neuromuscular junction disorders, 251, 261–272. *See also* Lambert-
Eaton myasthenic syndrome; Myasthenia gravis
botulism, 272
Neuronopathy, vs. neuropathy, 209
Neurosyphilis, 149–150
clinical syndromes of, 149
treatment of, 149–150
Night terrors, 241–242
Nightmares, 243
Nonsteroidal anti-inflammatory drugs, in prophylaxis of migraine, 198
Nystagmus, 18–19
in coma, 298
and vertigo, 26

Obstructive sleep apnea, 239
Ocular bobbing, in coma, 298
Ocular dipping, in coma, 298
Oculocephalic test, 298–299
Oculovestibular test, 26, 299
Olfactory nerve, examination of, 10–11
Optic neuritis. *See* Isolated idiopathic optic neuritis

Palmomental reflex, 43
Parasomnias, 240–244
   bruxism, 241
   enuresis, 240–241
   impaired or painful penile erection, 244
   nightmares, 243
   night terrors, 241–242
   periodic limb movements, 242
   post-traumatic stress disorder, 242
   rapid eye movement sleep disorder, 243
   restless legs syndrome, 242
   sinus cardiac arrest, 243
   sleep myoclonus, 242
   sleep talking, 241
   sleep walking, 241
Paratonia, 38
Paredrine test, 110
Parieto-occipital lobe lesion, 67
Parkinson's disease, 225–229
   clinical features of, 225–226
   differential diagnosis of, 226
   management of, 226–229
      pharmacotherapy, 228–229
      surgery, 229
Patrick's test, 55
Penile erection during sleep, impaired or painful, 244
Pergolide, in therapy of Parkinson's disease, 229
Perifascicular atrophy, 275
Periodic limb movements, 242
Peripheral neuropathy, 209–222, 255–261
   acute, 215–216
      mononeuropathies, 215–216, 218

acute peroneal nerve palsy, 215
acute radial nerve palsy, 215
acute seventh nerve (Bell's) palsy, 216, 255–256
acute third nerve palsy, 216
polyneuropathies, 74, 216, 218–219
diabetic, 259
causes of, 213–218
classification approach, 215–218
mnemonic approach, 214
clinical clues to, 221–222
electrophysiologic diagnosis of, 213
entrapment, 217–218, 220. *See also* Carpal tunnel syndrome;
Cubital tunnel syndrome
evaluation of, 209–210, 218–220
hereditary, 217, 219–220, 260–261
mononeuropathy multiplex, 217, 219
relapsing and remitting, 217, 219
signs of, 211–213
autonomic, 212
motor, 212
nail beds, 213
musculoskeletal, 213
palpable hypertrophic nerve, 212
skin lesions, 212–213
subacute, chronic, symmetric sensorimotor polyneuropathies,
216–217, 219
symptoms of, 210–211
autonomic, 211
motor, 211
sensory, 210–211
therapy for, 220–221
specific, 220–221
symptomatic, 221
Peroneal nerve palsy, acute, 215, 258–259
Persistent vegetative state, 293
Pharmacologic tests, 109–110
cocaine test, 109–110
edrophonium (Tensilon) test, 109
for myasthenia gravis, 262–263
Pharynx, examination of, 28

Phenytoin, in treatment of trigeminal neuralgia, 208
Pinprick test, 34
Plantar response, 41–42
Plasmapheresis
    in treatment of Guillain-Barré syndrome, 335
    in treatment of myasthenia gravis, 268
Plexopathies, 74–75
POEMS syndrome, 222
Polyneuropathies, 74, 251. *See also* Peripheral neuropathy
Polysomnogram, 99
Positive sharp waves, 90
Positron emission tomography, 86–87
Post-traumatic headache, 202
Post-traumatic stress disorder, 242
Posterior interosseus mononeuropathy, 75
Postsynaptic neuromuscular junction disorder, 77
Postural instability, in Parkinson's disease, 226
Pramipexole, in therapy of Parkinson's disease, 229
Prednisone, in treatment of temporal arteritis, 338–339
Presynaptic disorders, 270–272. *See also* Lambert-Eaton myasthenic
                syndrome
    botulism, 272
Primary muscle disease. *See* Myopathy
Primidone, for treatment of essential tremor, 230
Progressive multifocal leukoencephalopathy, 176
Pronator sign, 39, 55
Propranolol
    in prophylaxis of migraine, 198
    for treatment of essential tremor, 230
Protopathic pain, therapy for, 221
Pseudobulbar palsy, 24, 70
Pseudotumor cerebri, 203–204
    diagnostic tests for, 204–205
    eye symptoms in, 206
Ptosis, 12
Pupillary sparing, 56
Pupils
    abnormalities of
        Adie's pupil, 13

anisocoria, 13
  Argyll-Robertson pupils, 14
  Horner's syndrome, 13
  Marcus Gunn pupil, 13
in coma, 297
examination of, 12–14
comparison of dilation, 12
Pyridostigmine, for treatment of myasthenia gravis, 265, 266

Quadriceps, weakness and atrophy of, 77

Radial nerve lesions, 76
Radial nerve palsy, acute, 215
Radiculopathies, 74, 283–284, 288
Rapid eye movement sleep disorder, 243
Reflexes, 40–43
  corticobulbar, 43
  general rules for testing of, 40–41
  pathologic (frontal release signs), 43
  superficial, 41–42
    plantar, 41–42
Refsum's disease, 212, 215, 220, 221
Repetitive nerve stimulation test, in myasthenia gravis, 263
Respiratory patterns, in coma, 300–301
Restless legs syndrome, 242
Rigidity, 38
  definition of, 224–225
Riluzole, for treatment of amyotrophic lateral sclerosis, 254
Rinne test, 25
Rizatriptan, for treatment of migraine, 197
Romberg's test, 33
Ropinirole, in therapy of Parkinson's disease, 229

Scapular winging, 76
Scissoring gait, 45
Sclerosing panencephalitis, subacute, electroencephalography in, 98
Scopolamine disc, for symptoms of dizziness, 188
Seizures, 135–143. *See also* Epilepsy
  alcohol withdrawal, 180–181

Seizures (*continued*)
    definition of, 135
    differential diagnosis of, 135
    drug therapy for. *See* Antiepileptic drugs
    electroencephalography and, 136
    generalized, 137
    intractable, surgery for, 137
    partial, 136–137
      complex, 137
    in status epilepticus, 139
    vs. pseudoseizures, 140
    workup of unprovoked, 135
Selegiline, in therapy for Parkinson's disease, 228
Sensorineural hearing loss, 25
Sensory examination, 30–35
    anatomy, 30–31
    double simultaneous stimulation, 35
    pinprick test, 34
    screenings in, 31–32
    testing for joint position sense, 33–34
    testing for light touch, 32
    testing for temperature sensitivity, 34–35
    testing for vibration, 32–33
Sensory nerve action potential, measurement of, 89
Sensory nerve conduction studies, 89
Serotonin receptor agonists, for treatment of migraine, 196–197
Seventh nerve (Bell's) palsy, acute, 216, 255–256
Shoulders, examination of, 29–30
Single-photon emission computed tomography, 87–88
Sinus cardiac arrest, 243
Sleep
    biological rhythms and, 237
    cycles of, 236–237
    neuroanatomy and, 237
    non–rapid eye movement, 235–236
    rapid eye movement, 236
Sleep apnea syndrome, 239–240

Sleep disorders, 235–245
    diagnosis of, 244–245
    excessive daytime sleepiness (narcolepsy), 238–239
    insomnias, 237
    parasomnias, 240–244. *See also* Parasomnias
    sleep apnea syndrome, 239–240
    sleep-awake cycle disorders, 244
Sleep myoclonus, 242
Sleep studies, 99–100
Sleep talking, 241
Sleep walking, 241
Sleep-awake cycle disorders, 244
Snout reflex, 43
Somatosensory evoked potentials, 94–95
Spastic paraparesis, 69
Spasticity, 37
Spinal cord compression, metastatic epidural, 315–316
    evidence of, 286–287
Spinal cord lesion, hallmarks of, 71
Spinothalamic tract, 64
Sprain, muscle, 283
Status epilepticus, 139, 303–309
    in alcoholics, 181
    causes of, 303
    diagnosis of, 304
    electroencephalography in, 97, 308
    imaging in, 309
    key points about, 308–309
    management of, 304–308
        goals of therapy, 304–305
        follow-up and maintenance, 307
        guidelines for, 305
        steps of therapy for, 305–308
    prognosis in, 308
    refractory, 307
Status migrainosus, 198–199
Steppage, 45

Stereotactic thalamotomy, for treatment of essential tremor, 231
Sternomastoid muscle, weakness of, 29–30
Straight leg raising test, 55
Stroke, 113–133
   anterior circulation transient ischemic attacks and, 130
   anticoagulant therapy and, 131–132
   aphasia resulting from, 132–133
   causes of, in young adults, 129–130
   complications of, 119
   dissection as cause of, 127–128
   embolic, 123–124
   emergency room treatment of, 113–120
      initial assessment, 113–114
      further assessment, 116–117
         neurologic examination, 117
         neurovascular examination, 117
      management, 118–119
      therapeutic considerations, 114–116
         elevated blood pressure and, 114–116
      workup, 117–118
   lacunar, 122–123
   posterior circulation transient ischemic attacks and, 130–131
   prevention of, 120
   risk factors for, 119
Subarachnoid hemorrhage, 125–127
   causes of, 125
   eye symptoms in, 206
   imaging of, 126
   incidence of, 126
   treatment of, 126–127
Subcortical lesion, vs. parieto-occipital lobe lesion, 67
Sudomotor tests, 101
Sumatriptan, for treatment of migraine, 196
Supranuclear palsy, 19

Tardive dyskinesia, 232–233
   definition of, 224
Tarsal tunnel syndrome, 218
Temperature sensitivity, testing for, 34–35

Temporal arteritis, 337–339
    clinical presentation of, 337
    diagnostic tests for, 205, 337
    management of, 338–339
    diagnostic tests in, 205
Temporal artery biopsy, 107
Tensilon test, 109
    for myasthenia gravis, 262–263
Tension-type headache, 191
Theta waves, in electroencephalography, 95
Thiamine
    in delirium tremens, 322
    in Wernicke's encephalopathy, 326
Thiamine deficiency. *See* Wernicke's encephalopathy
Third nerve palsy, acute, 216
Thymectomy, in treatment of myasthenia gravis, 266–267, 269
Tiagabine, 143
Tics, definition of, 224
Tinel's sign, 54
Todd's paralysis, 56
Tolcapone, in therapy of Parkinson's disease, 229
Tolosa-Hunt syndrome, eye symptoms in, 207
Tongue
    deviation of, 73
    examination of, 27–28
Topiramate, 143
Touch, light, testing for, 32
Transcranial Doppler ultrasonography, 86
Transient ischemic attacks, 118, 120–122
    causes of, 121
    differential diagnosis of, 121
    risk factors for, 121
    treatment of, 122
    workup for, 118, 121
Transtentorial herniation, 312
    management of, 313–314
Transverse myelitis, acute, 174–175
    clinical features of, 174–175
    evaluation of, 175

Transverse myelitis, acute (*continued*)
  and multiple sclerosis, 175
  therapy for, 175
Trapezius, weakness of, 29–30, 76
Tremor, definition of, 224
Tricyclic antidepressants, in prophylaxis of migraine, 198
Trigeminal nerve, examination of, 20–22
  corneal reflex, 20–21
  jaw jerk, 20
  motor, 20
  sensation, 21–22
Trigeminal neuralgia, 207–208
  treatment of, 208
Trihexyphenidyl mesylate, in therapy of Parkinson's disease, 228
Trömner's reflex, 43
Truncal ataxia, 48
Tubular vision, 15

Uhthoff's phenomenon, 165
Ultrasonography, Doppler
  carotid, 85
  transcranial, 86
Uncal herniation, 312
Upper motor neuron weakness, 24

Vasculitis, central nervous system, 128–129
Verapamil, in prophylaxis of migraine, 198
Vertigo
  causes of, 184–187
    central nervous system, 185
    drugs, 185–186
    otologic, 186–187
  key points in history of patient with, 183
  key points in physical examination of patient with, 184
Vestibular exercise, in treatment of vertigo, 188
Vestibular neuronitis, 187
Vestibular system, examination of, 26
Vibration, testing for, 32–33

Vigabatrin, 143
Visual acuity, examination of, 14
Visual evoked potentials, 93
Visual field, examination of, 14–15
Visual inattention, 14
Visual tract (straight), 65

Waddling gait, 45
Wallenberg's syndrome, 69
Watershed infarcts, 68
Weber's test, 25
Wernicke's encephalopathy, 325–327
    clinical features of, 325
    common mistakes in treatment of, 327
    diagnosis of, 326
    management of, 326
Withdrawal response, 42
Wrist extensors, strength of
Wristdrop, 75–76

X-rays, 81

Zolmitriptan, for treatment of migraine, 196–197